A PAEDIATRIC VADE-MECUM

PRINCIPAL CONTRIBUTORS

NEETA M. BAMPTON, B. PHARM., M.P.S.

P. R. BETTS, M.B., B.S., M.R.C.P.

M. J. BRUETON, M.B., B.S., M.R.C.P., D.C.H.

ANNE DE LOOY, B.SC., PH.D., S.R.D.

R. H. GEORGE, M.B., CH.B., M.R.C.PATH.

J. INSLEY, M.B., F.R.C.P.

JILLIAN R. MANN, M.B., B.S., M.R.C.P.

D. N. RAINE, M.B., B.SC., PH.D.

B. A. WHARTON, M.D., F.R.C.P., D.C.H.

A Paediatric Vade-Mecum

EDITED BY

BEN WOOD
D.M., F.R.C.P.

Consultant Paediatrician, United Birmingham Hospitals and Birmingham Regional Hospital Board

Ninth Edition

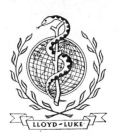

LLOYD-LUKE (MEDICAL BOOKS) LTD
49 NEWMAN STREET
LONDON
1977

First six editions published by the
United Birmingham Hospitals

SEVENTH EDITION	..	..	1970
Italian Translation	..	..	1971
Reprinted	..	..	..	1972
French Translation	..	..	1973
EIGHTH EDITION	..	..	..	1974
Greek Translation	..	..	1976
NINTH EDITION	..	..	..	1977

PRINTED AND BOUND IN ENGLAND BY
THE WHITEFRIARS PRESS LTD. LONDON AND TONBRIDGE

ISBN 0 85324 126 0

FOREWORD

This is the ninth edition of the Birmingham *Paediatric Vademecum*, and the third to be edited by Dr Ben Wood. Of the nine principal contributors to the present book, six are new. Dr Wood selects his contributors skilfully and manages them deftly. Each edition of the book has been better than its predecessor and it is now widely appreciated in Britain and in three other European countries. It is valued, not only by "hard-pressed house persons" (Wood), but also by junior staff, paediatricians and general practitioners, and by all those who seek its help in the medical care of children.

This handbook provides the essential facts of development, nutrition and clinical chemistry, together with advice on the management and treatment of the most important disorders, diseases and emergencies of childhood. There are also comprehensive and lucid instructions on the use of nearly 200 drugs. Accuracy, clarity and brevity have obviously been the editorial watchwords.

How fortunate then are the doctors who will read this book and assimilate its advice. Their professional consciences will be untroubled and their sleep be undisturbed, except for the practice of good paediatrics. If they find that their heads cannot contain all its information, the book itself will fit snugly into the pockets of their white coats.

DOUGLAS HUBBLE, K.B.E., M.D., F.R.C.P.
Emeritus Professor of Paediatrics
University of Birmingham

EDITOR'S NOTE

Once again I must thank the many colleagues who gave their time and knowledge to this new edition. In particular I must mention Drs. Jenny Edwards, Peter Jeavons, Brian Rudd, Eric Silove, Richard White and Mr. Douglas Jackson.

"S.I." units are now widely used if not totally accepted, but we continue to give both values although it may prolong the agony.

The chapters on nutrition, fluids and electrolytes have been completely re-written in the light of recent changes in available milk preparations. Other new or expanded sections include infantile gastro-enteritis, thyroid function tests, fits in childhood, and reporting deaths to the Coroner.

We have included a rather complex table on digoxin dosage (p. 105) because deaths and near-deaths from a misplaced decimal point still occur. Nearly everyone has his own individual method of calculating digoxin dosage: all we suggest is that after so doing, they check on page 105 to see that they are not giving ten or a hundred times too much. For a similar reason a rough guide to rehydration is placed amongst the theoretical calculations (p. 51) for the benefit of hard-pressed house persons trying to work out arithmetic in the small hours.

BEN WOOD

May 1977

CONTENTS

FOREWORD   v

EDITOR'S NOTE   vii

I   NORMAL DATA   1

Normal Development in Infancy and Childhood, 5
Warning Signs at Different Ages, 7
Chronological Order of Appearance and Union of Osseous Centres, 8
Centiles of Height, Weight and Skull Circumference, 11

II   NUTRITION   15

Healthy Children: Daily Intake and Milk Formulae, 17
Sick Children: Tube Feeding, 21
Common Nutritional Problems, 23
Other Disorders, 26
Special Feeds, Diets and Supplements, 29

III   FLUID AND ELECTROLYTE THERAPY   45

Maintenance Requirements, 47
Replacement of Deficit and Correction of Losses, 48
Rough Guide to Rehydration, 51
Parenteral Nutrition, 52

IV   THE NEWBORN   57

General Care at Birth, 59
Examination of the Newborn, 60
Special Problems, 63
Major Symptoms, 65
Haemolytic Disease of the Newborn, 71
Neonatal Infections, 73

V   INFECTIONS   75

    Pyrexia of Uncertain Origin, 77
    Table of Incubation and Isolation, 78
    Worm, Protozoal and Candidal Infections, 79
    Virus Infections, Vaccinia, Herpes, 82
    Suggested Immunisation Schedule, 84
    Tetanus Prophylaxis, 85

VI   PAEDIATRIC EMERGENCIES   87

    Dehydration, Infantile Gastro-enteritis, 89
    Convulsions and Coma, 90
    Respiratory Emergencies, 91
    Acute Collapse in Infancy, 94
    Adrenocortical Crisis, 95
    Acute Renal Failure, 96
    Diabetes Mellitus, 100
    Congenital Heart Lesions and Cardiac
    Emergencies, Digoxin Dosage, 103
    Burns, 109

VII   ACCIDENTAL POISONING   111

    Poison Information Centres, 113
    Initial Management, 113
    Specific Poisons: Salicylates, Iron, Psychotropic
       Drugs, Tricyclic Antidepressants, Atropine
       Group, Amphetamine, Alcohol, Household
       Products, Caustic Burns, Paraffin, Paraquat
       and Diquat, Plants, Lead, 115

VIII   DIAGNOSIS AND MANAGEMENT OF   123
       HAEMATOLOGICAL DISORDERS

    Leukaemia, 125
    Haemorrhagic Disorders, 127
    Haemoglobinopathies, 129
    G-6-PD Deficiency, 130
    Coagulation Investigations, 132
    Routine Haematological Values, 133

IX   CLINICAL CHEMISTRY   135

    Average Biochemical Standards, 137
    Acid-Base Balance, 139

Glucose Tolerance, 139
Hypoglycaemia, 140
Pituitary, Adrenal and Gonadal Function, 141
Thyroid Function, 143
Renal Function, 144
Special Tests, 146
Gastro-intestinal Function, 147

X   MISCELLANEOUS   151

Management of Children with Non-accidental
    Injuries, 153
Nuclear Sexing and Chromosomal Analysis,
    155
Genetic Counselling, 155
Amniocentesis, 156
Fits in Childhood, 157
Reporting Deaths to the Coroner, 159

XI   PAEDIATRIC PRESCRIBING   165

Notes for Prescribers, 167
Calculation of Dosage for Children, 167
Nomogram for Estimating Surface Area, 168
Some Important Drugs, 171

XII   ANTIBIOTIC AND CHEMOTHERAPY   185

General Considerations, 187
Principal Antibiotic and Chemotherapeutic
    Agents, 189
Usual Sensitivity Pattern of Some Bacteria, 193
Antibiotics and the Blood-Brain Barrier, 194

XIII   CORTICOSTEROIDS   195

General Considerations, 197
Precautions in Treatment, 197
Outpatient Care, 198
Principal Steroids and Dosage, 199

INDEX   201

I
NORMAL DATA

NORMAL DATA

The assessment of mental and physical development depends on statistics based mainly on normal Caucasian children. Allowance must therefore be made for race, environment, intra-uterine growth and gestation.

The following table should be interpreted in this light and corrections should be made for gestational or conceptual age as described in Chapter IV.

Development Assessment

The first table on normal development deals with children up to 2 years. Beyond this age Professor Illingworth's and Dr. Sheridan's books should be consulted. The second table gives some of the more important warning signs in infants seen at predetermined ages. If the infant shows any of these signs appropriate investigation is indicated.

The references below provide further information on this and related subjects.

Physical Growth

The tables for weight, height and skull circumference give an indication of the percentile status at the time of examination; for long-term observation of the individual child suitable charts are available as shown below.

REFERENCES

EGAN, D. F., ILLINGWORTH, R. S., and MACKEITH, R. C. (1969). *Developmental Screening 0 to 5 Years*. London: Spastics Medical Publications.

GRIFFITHS, M. I. (1973). *The Young Retarded Child*. London: Churchill Livingstone.

GRIFFITHS, RUTH (1954). *The Abilities of Babies*. London: University of London Press.

ILLINGWORTH, R. S. (1975). *The Development of the Infant and Young Child*, 6th edit. Edinburgh: Churchill Livingstone.

SHERIDAN, MARY D. (1975). *The Developmental Progress of Infants and Young Children*, 3rd edit. London: H.M.S.O.

CHARTS

Height, length, weight charts from 28 weeks gestation to 100 weeks, by Gairdner, D., and Pearson, J. Printed by Creasey's, Bull Lane, Hertfordshire.

Growth and Development record, by Tanner, J. M., and White-house, R. H. Printed by Printwell Press Ltd., Bristow Works, Bristow Road, Hounslow, Middlesex.

NORMAL DEVELOPMENT IN INFANCY AND CHILDHOOD

Age in Months*	Motor	Social	Hearing and Speech	Eye and Hand
1	Head erect for few seconds	Quieted when picked up	Startled by sounds	Follows light with eyes
2	Head up when prone (chin clear)	Smiles	Listens to bell or rattle	Follows ring up, down and sideways
3	Kicks well	Follows person with eyes	Searches for sound with eyes	Glances from one object to another
4	Lifts head and chest prone	Returns examiner's smile	Laughs	Clasps and retains cube
5	Holds head erect with no lag	Frolics when played with	Turns head to sound	Pulls paper away from face
6	Rises on to wrists	Turns head to person talking	Babbles or coos to voice or music	Takes cube from table
7	Rolls from front to back	Drinks from a cup	Makes four different sounds	Looks for fallen objects
8	Sits without support	Looks at mirror image	Understands "No" and "Bye Bye"	Passes toy from hand to hand
9	Turns around on floor	Helps to hold cup for drinking	Says "Mama" or "Dada"	Manipulates two objects together
10	Stands when held up	Smiles at mirror image	Imitates playful sounds	Clicks two objects together in imitation.
11	Pulls up to stand	Finger feeds	Two words with meaning	Pincer grip
12	Walks or side-steps around pen	Plays pat-a-cake on request	Three words with meaning	Finds toy hidden under cup

NORMAL DEVELOPMENT IN INFANCY AND CHILDHOOD—(Continued)

Age in Months	Motor	Social	Hearing and Speech	Eye and Hand
13	Stands alone	Holds cup for drinking	Looks at pictures	Preference for one hand
14	Walks alone	Uses spoon	Recognises own name	Makes marks with pencil
15	Climbs up stairs	Shows shoes	Four to five clear words	Places one object upon another
16	Pushes pram, toy horse, etc.	Tries to turn door knob	Six to seven clear words	Scribbles freely
17	Picks up toy from floor without falling	Manages cup well	Babbled conversation	Pulls (table) cloth to get toy
18	Climbs on to chair	Takes off shoes and socks	Enjoys rhymes and tries to join in	Constructive play with toys
19	Climbs stairs up and down	Knows one part of the body	Nine words	Tower of three bricks
20	Jumps	Bowel control	Twelve words	Tower of four bricks
21	Runs	Bladder control by day	Two-word sentences	Circular scribble
22	*Walks* up stairs	Tries to tell experiences	Listens to stories	Tower of five or more bricks
23	Seats himself at table	Knows two parts of body	Twenty words or more	Copies perpendicular stroke
24	*Walks* up and down stairs	Knows four parts of body	*Names* four toys	Copies horizontal stroke

*Conceptual rather than chronological age.

WARNING SIGNS AT DIFFERENT AGES

Age*	Weight (kg) 3rd–97th centiles	Skull Circ. (cm)	General	Hearing and Speech	Vision	Arms	Legs	Pelvis
6 weeks	3·4/5·9	35/41	Any major maternal anxiety. "Fits", "spasms", or "colic" of uncertain origin at any time especially first six months.	Absence of auditory "alertness"	Lack of fixation or following at 9–12 in. distance. Cataract	Excessive head lag on pulling to sitting position. Asymmetry in movements, tone or neonatal responses	Immobility or undue extension	Definite click or instability of hips. Absent femoral pulses.
6 months	5·9/9·4	40/45	Persistence of heart murmur. Lack of smiling. Fits or spasms as above. Persistence of hand regard	Failure to localise to soft sound on either side	Failure to fix and follow both near and far objects around 180°. Persistent squint	Failure to reach out or transfer (both hands). Persistent fisting or preference for one hand	Increased adductor tone. Increased reflexes. Clonus	Limited abduction of hips. (X-ray if necessary)
10 months	7·2/11·0	43/49	Absence of chewing. Lack of imitation	Absence of babble	Squint or nystagmus	Abnormal hand posture or ataxia	Absence of weight bearing whilst held	Failure to sit without support
18 months	8·8/13·6	45/50	Absence of constructive play. Persistence of casting drooling or mouthing	Lack of spontaneous vocalisation	Any apparent visual defect	Abnormal grasp, abnormal hand posture, no pincer grip	Inability to stand without support	
2 years	9·6/14·9	46/51	Hyperkinesia, failure to concentrate.	Absence of recognisable words	Failure to match toys	Tremor or ataxia with bricks	Lack of walking without aid	

*Conceptual rather than chronological age.

CHRONOLOGICAL ORDER OF APPEARANCE OF OSSEOUS CENTRES

	BIRTH	1 YEAR	2	3	4	5
Shoulder 0	Head of humerus (3 mths.)	Great tuberosity				
Elbow 0		Capitellum				Head of radius
Hand 0	Hamate (4 mths.) Capitate (6 mths.) Ep. radius		Triquet-rum Ep. meta-carpals Ep. phalanges	Lunatum	Trapez-ium Scaphoid
Hip 0	Head of femur (9 mths.)			Great troch-anter	
Knee Ep. femur and tibia				Head of fibula	Patella
Foot Cuboid	Ext. cuneiform Ep. tibia	Ep. fibia	Int. cuneiform Ep. meta-tarsals	Mid cuneiform Navicular	

The new centres of ossification which appear at each year are shown in black. From Lawson Wilkins, *The Diagnosis and Treatment of Endocrine Disorders in Childhood and Adolescence* (3rd edit., 1965).
Courtesy of Charles C. Thomas, Publisher, Springfield, Illinois.

CHRONOLOGICAL ORDER OF APPEARANCE OF UNION OF EPIPHYSIS WITH DIAPHYSIS

6	7	8	9	10	11 yrs.
Union head and tuberosity					
Int. epicondyle			Trochlea Olecranon		Ext. epicondyle
Trapezoid Ep. ulna				Pisiform	
	Union ischium & pubis			Ep. lesser trochanter	
					Tibial tubercle
		Ep. os calcis			

The new centres of ossification which appear at each year are shown in black. From Lawson Wilkins, *The Diagnosis and Treatment of Endocrine Disorders in Childhood and Adolescence* (3rd edit., 1965).

Courtesy of Charles C. Thomas, Publisher, Springfield, Illinois.

CHRONOLOGICAL ORDER OF UNION OF EPIPHYSIS WITH DIAPHYSIS

Years	12	13	14	15	17	18
Shoulder						Head of humerus Great tuberosity
Elbow	Trochlea and capitellum	Olecranon	Ext. epicondyle Head of radius			
Hand				Ep. metacarpals and phalanges		Ep. radius and ulna
Hip				Head of femur Trochanters		
Knee						Ep. femur tibia and fibula
Foot				Ep. metatarsals and phalanges	Ep. tibia and fibula	

From Lawson Wilkins, *The Diagnosis and Treatment of Endocrine Disorders in Childhood and Adolescence* (3rd edit., 1965). Courtesy of Charles C. Thomas, Publisher, Springfield, Illinois.

CENTILE TABLE FOR BOYS

Gestation weeks	Weight kg			Height cm*			Skull Circumference cm*		
	10	50	90	10	50	90	10	50	90
28	0·8	1·1	1·4	36	38	40	25	26	27·5
30	1·1	1·5	2·0	38·5	40·5	42	27	28	29·5
32	1·5	2·0	2·6	41	43	44·5	28·5	30	31
34	2·0	2·5	3·2	43	45	47	30	31·5	33
36	2·4	3·0	3·6	45	47	49	31·5	33	34
38	2·6	3·3	3·9	47	48·5	51	32·5	34	35·5
40	2·9	3·5	4·2	48	50	53	33·5	35	36·5
Age	3	50	97	3	50	97	3	50	97
3 months	4·4	5·7	7·2	55	60	65	38	41	43
6 months	6·2	7·8	9·8	62	66·5	71	41	44	46
9 months	7·6	9·3	11·6	66·5	71	76	43	46	47
12 months	8·4	10·3	12·8	70	75	80	44	47	49
18 months	9·4	11·7	14·2	75	81	87	46	49	51
2 years	10·2	12·7	15·7	80	87	93	47	50	52
3 years	11·6	14·7	17·8	86	95	102	48	50	53
4 years	13	15	21	94	101	110			
5 years	14	19	23	100	108	117	49	51	54
6 years	16	21	27	105	114	124			
7 years	17	23	30	110	120	130			
8 years	19	25	34	115	126	137	50	52	55
9 years	21	27·5	39	120	132	143			
10 years	23	30	44	125	137	148			
11 years	25	34	50	129	142	154			
12 years	27	38	58	133	147	160	51	54	56
13 years	30	43	64	138	153	168			
14 years	33	49	71	144	160	176	53	56	58
15 years	39	55	76	152	167	182			
16 years	46	60	79	158	172	185			
17 years	49	62	80	162	174	187			
18 years	50	64	82	162	175	187			

* To nearest half cm.

CENTILE TABLE FOR GIRLS

Gestation weeks	Weight kg			Height cm*			Skull Circumference cm*		
	10	50	90	10	50	90	10	50	90
28	0·75	1·1	1·5	36·5	38	40	25	26	27·5
30	1·0	1·5	2·1	38·5	40·5	42	27	28	29·5
32	1·5	2·0	2·7	41	43	44·5	28·5	30	31·0
34	1·8	2·5	3·3	43	45	47	30	31·5	33
36	2·3	2·8	3·6	45	47	49	31·5	33	34
38	2·6	3·2	3·8	47	48·5	51	32·5	34	35·5
40	2·8	3·4	4·0	48	49	52	33·5	35	36
Age	3	50	97	3	50	97	3	50	97
3 months	4·2	5·2	7·0	55	58	62	37	40	43
6 months	5·9	7·3	9·4	61	65	69	40	43	45
9 months	7·0	8·7	10·9	65	70	74	42	44	47
12 months	7·6	9·6	12·0	69	74	78	43	46	48
18 months	8·8	10·9	13·6	75	80	85	45	47	50
2 years	9·6	12·0	14·9	79	85	91	46	48	51
3 years	11·2	14·1	17·4	86	93	100	47	49	52
4 years	13	16	20	92	100	109			
5 years	15	18	23	98	107	116	48	50	53
6 years	16	20	27	104	114	123			
7 years	18	23	30	109	120	130			
8 years	19	25	35	114	125	136	50	52	54
9 years	21	28	40	120	130	142			
10 years	23	31	48	125	136	148			
11 years	25	35	56	130	143	155			
12 years	28	40	64	135	149	164	51	53	56

CENTILE TABLE FOR GIRLS—*continued*

Gestation weeks	Weight kg			Height cm*			Skull Circumference cm*		
	10	**50**	**90**	**10**	**50**	**90**	**10**	**50**	**90**
13 years	32	46	70	142	156	168			
14 years	37	51	73	148	160	172	52	54	57
15 years	42	54	74	150	162	173			
16 years	45	56	75	151	162	174			
17 years	46	56	75	—	—	—			
18 years	46	57	75	—	—	—			

* To nearest half cm.

From Gairdner, D., and Pearson, J. (1971), *Arch. Dis. Childh.*, **46,** 783; and Tanner, J. M., Whitehouse, R. H., and Takaishi, M. (1966) *Arch. Dis. Childh.*, **41,** 454.

Adapted from Westrop, C. K., and Barber, C. R. (1956), *J. Neurol., Neurosurg. Psychiat.*, **19,** 52.

B.W.

II
NUTRITION

A guide to advisable intakes of nutrients is given in Table I.

Younger Infant (Birth till weaning).

Breast feeding. Antenatal preparation is important in promotion of breast feeding. The baby receives colostrum which is rich in trace elements and anti-infective factors during the first two days of breast feeding after which mature milk "comes in". Thereafter the baby may wish to feed as often as two-hourly but more usually 3- or 4-hourly. Successful breast feeding ensures close contact between mother and child and minimises the risk of bacterial contamination of the milk. Breast milk itself has advantages over unmodified cow's milk in that the concentrations of protein, phosphorus and major minerals are lower, the fat is more easily absorbed, quality of the protein may be more suitable in the early days of life and it contains anti-infective substances, e.g. lactoferrin and maternal IgA. Vitamin supplements are recommended for breast-fed infants (7 drops daily of the DHSS mixture—see p. 20).

Bottle feeding.—Feeding usually commences during first 12 hours of life and continues every 3–4 hours thereafter, eventually missing out the night feed to give *approximately* a 4-hourly, 5 times a day, regular, but flexible, routine. One of the formulae shown in Table II is recommended. It is fed to satisfy appetite which will be approximately 150 ml per kg per day (120–180 ml) during the first 4 months of life. This will supply all the necessary nutrients, but vitamin supplements are currently recommended for all babies (see p. 20). Great care is needed in reconstitution of the feeds, e.g. cleaning and sterilising of bottles, teats, etc., measuring of fluid and scoops of powder, particularly to avoid too concentrated feeds, and handling of feed after reconstitution to avoid bacterial growth.

Older Infant (Weaning till first birthday)

Mixed feeding should start between 4 and 6 months. Too early introduction of mixed feeding may contribute to renal osmolar load problems, obesity in Britain, undernutrition in developing countries, and development of coeliac disease in the young infant. Too late introduction might (theoretically)

TABLE I
Daily Intakes in Healthy Children

	Younger[a] infant	Older infant	Toddler	Primary schoolchild	Secondary schoolchild
Age (years)	0–5/12	6–11/12	1–4	5–11	12–18
	Intake per kg body wt	Total intake per day			
Energy					
MJ	0·430	3·8–4·2	5–7	7–10	10–13
kcal	100	910–1000	12–1600	18–2400	25–3000
Protein (g)	1·5	23–25	30–40	45–60	60–75
Vitamins					
A (retinol μg)	90	150	300	300–600	750
Thiamine mg	0·03	0·2	0·6	0·7–1·0	1·0
Nicotinic acid mg	1	5	7–9	10–14	16–19
C mg	6	20	20	25	30
D (chole-calciferol μg)	5[b]	10	10	2·5	2·5
Sodium mmol	1·0	6[c]	8[c]	50[c]	100[c]
Potassium mmol	2·3	6	8	20	50
Magnesium mmol	0·2	1·0	1·0	10	15
Calcium mmol	1·3	9	13	13–18	18
Iron mmol	0·002	0·1	0·15	0·2	0·25
Water litres [d]	0·12–0·18	0·8–1·2	1–1·5	1–1·5	1·2–1·5

Notes: (a) Figures for younger infant are those contained in 150 ml of human milk.
(b) As vitamin D sulphate.
(c) Electrolytes in older infants and toddlers mainly from Fomon (1974) *Infant Nutrition* (Philadelphia: W. B. Saunders). Much higher intakes are common, but are not necessary; in schoolchildren figures are based on observed intakes.
(d) This does not include water found in solid food; a fully mixed diet may contribute the same volume of water again; total water requirements are related to energy and solute content of diet.

Other figures mainly from DHSS (1974) *Recommended Intakes of Nutrients.*

Atomic weights: Sodium 23, Potassium 39, Magnesium 24, Calcium 40, Iron 56. Energy value of nutrients (kJ per g): protein 17, carbohydrate 16, fat 37. 1 MJ = 240 kcal. 1 kcal = 4·2 kJ.

TABLE II
ANALYSIS OF MILK FORMULAE (PER LITRE RECONSTITUTED FEED)

	Energy MJ (kcal)	Protein g	Fat g	Carbohydrate g	Vitamin A µg (a) retinol	Vitamin C mg	Vitamin D µg (b) calciferol	Sodium mmol	Potassium mmol	Magnesium mmol	Calcium mmol	Phosphorus mmol	Iron mmol
Suitable for younger and older infants													
Human milk	2·8 (690)	10	42	74	600	38	0·1 (c)	7	15	1·2	9	5	0·01
Cow and Gate Plus	2·6 (630)	18	33 (d)	66	1000	53	11	13	18	—	16	16	0·1
V Formula	2·6 (620)	18	30 (d)	70	790	53	11	14	21	2·2	16	16	0·1
Premium	2·6 (630)	18 (e)	33 (d)	69	790	50	11	10	15	2·0	14	13	0·1
Ostermilk Complete	2·7 (650)	17	27	86 (f)	1050	64	10	13	21	2·5	14	15	0·2
SMA	2·7 (650)	15 (e)	35 (d)	70	800	53	11	11	19	2·3	13	14	0·2
Gold Cap SMA-S26	2·8 (670)	15 (e)	36 (d)	72	800	53	11	7	14	2·0	11	11	0·1
New Ostermilk Two	2·6 (630)	18 (e)	25	83 (g)	1050	63	10	13	21	2·5	14	15	0·1
New Osterfeed	2·8 (680)	15 (e)	38	70	1040	69	10	7	15	2·0	9	10	0·1
Doorstep cow's milk	2·8 (660)	33	37	48	400	16	0·6	25	36	5·0	31	31	0·02

Notes:
(a) 1 µg retinol = 3·3 iu vitamin A.
(b) 1 µg cholecalciferol = 40 units vitamin D.
(c) Recent analyses suggest higher content as vitamin D sulphate.
(d) Contains vegetable and animal oils other than cow's milk fat.
(e) Modified cow's milk protein, curd : whey protein ratio similar to human milk.
(f) Approximately 30 g lactose, rest maltodextrins (hydrolysed starch).
(g) Approximately 53 g lactose, rest maltodextrins.

lead to deficiency of trace elements and (if on unmodified cow's milk) essential fatty acids or refusal to chew and swallow solid food.

A teaspoonful of baby rice mixed with water or milk may be given before a milk feed and the amount gradually increased. Other foods (commercially available or home prepared) are then introduced, such as broth, mixed sieved vegetables, mashed potatoes and gravy, milk puddings, fish, minced meat, etc., and up to 600 ml of milk should be continued throughout infancy.

After introducing mixed feeding, breast feeding or one of the formulae shown in Table II may be continued, or doorstep milk may be substituted. If doorstep milk is used, vitamin supplements are essential (see below) and because of the high renal solute load of doorstep milk the infant will probably want extra water. In developing countries breast feeding should be encouraged for many months after introducing mixed feeding, well into the second year of life.

Vitamin supplements.—Seven drops (0·2 ml) of the British DHSS vitamin drops contain vitamin A 300 µg as retinol (1000 iu), vitamin C 30 mg and vitamin D 10 µg (calciferol 400 iu); the recommended doses are:

age 1–4 months   4 drops (breast fed), 2 drops (formula fed)

age over 4 months   7 drops (breast fed or on doorstep milk), 4 drops (formula fed)

This supplementation is not essential for the formula-fed baby, but the total intakes of the potentially dangerous vitamins A and D from the formulae and supplements together are not excessive and help to establish the habit with the mother in case she later uses doorstep milk, when full supplements are essential.

The need for supplements in other countries is variable.

Toddlers (1–4-year-olds)

By his first birthday the British child is usually eating three or four meals a day, preferably with other members of the family and from the same menu. Many children will continue to drink up to 500 ml of doorstep milk during their toddler years and this provides a substantial proportion of their intake of protein (18 g), calcium (15 mmol) and riboflavine (700 µg).

A few drink very little milk, however, with no obvious ill-health. Many mothers become worried by an apparently poor appetite, food fads, and a lack of variety in the foods accepted by the child at this age. Comparing the child's weight and height to growth charts usually shows that they are normal and nutritional analysis of many of these diets, which at first glance seem of limited value, often shows them to be quite adequate. Reassurance that the child will grow out of these food fads is often all that is required. However, some children who truly have a low energy consumption are lighter than average and a few who present with short stature in Britain at this age have a limited and capricious diet. They may require further investigation.

Obesity may develop at this age or during the school years and some remain obese in adult life. Many children who were obese in late infancy are no longer so by the age of school entry.

In developing countries, however, mortality rates in toddlers are sometimes 30 times higher than in Britain due mainly to the combined effects of protein-energy malnutrition and infection.

Schoolchildren

In Britain early school years are usually nutritionally stable. The increased growth velocity during adolescence rarely imposes any nutritional strain but rickets and goitre may occur occasionally and menarche is later in undernourished girls. British school meals aim to provide one-third of the recommended daily intake of energy and one-third to half of the protein. Free school meals and milk are available for certain children.

Pellagra may occur in South African children at this age and a syndrome of hypogonadism and short stature probably due to zinc deficiency occurs in Persian boys.

SICK CHILDREN

Infancy

The regime described for mild gastro-enteritis (see p. 89) is also suitable for the feverish anorexic infant with, e.g., respiratory tract, or urinary tract infection. During this temporary period of higher fluid losses the aim is to give extra "free" water, reintroducing the normal diet gradually. Wherever possible breast feeding should continue during the illness to maintain lactation—particularly in developing countries.

Older Children

The aim is to maintain the advisable fluid intake (see Table I, p. 18) and to encourage the child to take an extra amount (2–5 per cent of body weight is a guide) if he is pyrexial, dyspnoeic or has loose stools. The choice of fluid is largely dictated by what the child will take. Mineral waters, tea, milk, etc., are all suitable, but the mineral waters and milk are preferably diluted with some water to reduce the sugar content. Ice lollipops, ice cream and jellies are a useful way of giving extra water. Solid foods are reintroduced after a few days as appetite returns.

FLUID DIET TO GIVE BY MOUTH, BY INTRAGASTRIC TUBE OR INTRAJEJUNAL TUBE

These diets are suitable for a child who has near normal gastro-intestinal, metabolic, cardiac and renal function, but who cannot take food normally, e.g. in coma, prolonged anorexia, abnormalities of nasopharynx and oesophagus.

Young infant.—The formulae recommended for the young infant (see p. 19) may all be given by tube.

Older infant, toddler and schoolchild.—When tube feeding is required for a short period (10 days or less) a simple mixture shown in Table III may be used.

Tube Feeding Technique

To pass an *intragastric* tube, the distance from nose to xiphisternum is marked on the tube; the tube is moistened with water and then gently pushed into the nose of the child—pushing backwards rather than upwards—until the mark is reached. To confirm that the tube is in the stomach inject a few ml of air down the tube while listening for the "gurgle" over the epigastrium with a stethoscope. If in place secure the tube to the child's cheek with adhesive tape. If the tube is of polyvinyl, or similar material, it may remain *in situ* for about a week. Feeds should be given about every 3 hours to young infants, more frequently to low birth weight babies, and less frequently to older children.

TABLE III
Fluid Diet Formula

Ingredients	Nutritional value per litre of feed	
Doorstep milk 800 ml	Protein	26 g
Prosparol or Double Cream 50 ml	Fat	55 g
Sucrose or Caloreen 60 g	Carbohydrate	98 g
Tap water, make up to 1 litre	Energy	4·1 MJ (990 kcal)
	Sodium	20 mmol
	Magnesium	4 mmol
	Potassium	29 mmol
	Calcium	25 mmol

1. Give sufficient to meet energy requirements shown in Table I (p. 18) or as an alternative rule after the first birthday give 1200 ml of the mixture, plus an extra 100 ml for each year of age up to a maximum of 2½ litres, e.g. 3-year-old—1500 ml, 15-year-old—2500 ml.
2. Give Abidec 0·6 ml daily.
3. For longer term, note that this diet is high in calcium and deficient in iron.

A *nasojejunal* tube is passed into the stomach as above and then allowed to pass by peristalsis into the duodenum or jejunum. Experience with this technique is still limited, but feeds should be given at least 2-hourly and possibly by continuous drip.

COMMON PRIMARY NUTRITIONAL DISORDERS IN BRITAIN

Obesity

"Simple" obesity is usually associated with increased height and bone age—retardation in either suggests the obesity is part of some other syndrome. Treatment is difficult, amounting to dietary restriction only; prevention is therefore preferable.

Simple reducing diet.—In severe cases, admission to hospital may be required and 1·5 MJ (359 kcals) given. A diet of 3–4 MJ (718–957 kcals) is more suitable for outpatient treatment. These energy intakes are sufficiently low for the treatment of obesity in both toddlers and schoolchildren.

1. No fried foods nor foods containing high proportions of fats, e.g. chips, pastry, cream, oil, salad creams. No sugar nor sugar-containing foods, e.g. cakes, sweets of all kinds, fizzy pop, tinned fruits and puddings.

2. *Allowed daily:*—15 g butter or margarine, three servings of lean meat or fish (white), or cottage cheese or egg—each not to exceed 60 g. 40 g of cheese allowed three times a week.

3. *Free foods allowed:*—Saccharine (no other sweetener). Diabetic fruit squash and pastilles (no other diabetic products). Salad vegetables and all green vegetables, except peas. Grapefruit, rhubarb and gooseberries—no sugar.

4. Carbohydrate-containing foods allowed as exchangeable portions from following list. The number of portions allowed will indicate the degree of energy restriction:

7 portions (i.e. 70 g carbohydrate) = 3 MJ total energy intake per day.

10 portions (i.e. 100 g carbohydrate) = 4·2 MJ total energy intake per day.

Exchangeable portions (10 g) of carbohydrate:

One thin slice off small loaf (20 g), 2 thin slices Procea or 2 crispbreads or 2 water biscuits, 15 g unsweetened breakfast cereal or other dry cereal, e.g. rice, macaroni, 15 g plain biscuits, e.g. Marie or Rich Tea, 200 ml (1 glass) milk, 60 g boiled potato, 60 g baked beans, 120 g fresh or frozen peas, 60 g tinned or processed peas, 90 g parsnips, 120 g fresh (or stewed without sugar) apple, pear, orange, or fruit juice, unsweetened, 60 g banana.

An extensive list of 10 g portions is available from the British Diabetic Association.

Scurvy

This can occur in late infancy but is now very rare in Britain. The child may present with bleeding gums, fine purpura or a pseudo-paralysis due to subperiosteal haemorrhage.

Treatment: ascorbic acid orally 500 mg once, then 100 mg daily for one week, then prophylactic dose 30 mg daily.

Prevention: see Vitamin Supplements, page 20.

Rickets

In Britain, Asian infants and adolescents, and older infants receiving doorstep milk without vitamins, may develop rickets.

Other causes of rickets, e.g. anticonvulsant therapy, malabsorption, renal glomerular and tubular disease and hypophosphatasia are much rarer causes, but must be considered particularly in a child not in one of the above groups.

Treatment in infancy: Vitamin D (calciferol) orally, 75 µg (3000 units) daily until healing of bones has occurred and serum alkaline phosphatase is normal, then prophylactic dose 10 µg (100 units) daily. In developing countries where daily treatment may be difficult, a single I.M. dose of 1500 µg (60,000 units) calciferol may be given.

This regime will cure primary nutritional rickets and that due to malabsorption or anticonvulsants; it will not cover up instances of renal glomerular or tubular rickets.

Prevention: see Vitamin Supplements, page 20.

Iron Deficiency Anaemia

Preterm babies, twins, older infants in whom weaning has been delayed, and toddlers who dislike meat or vegetables, often develop iron deficiency anaemia. The possibility of blood loss, particularly from the gastro-intestinal tract should be considered; malabsorption may present this way, and sometimes apparent iron deficiency anaemia is really thalassaemia or lead poisoning.

Treatment: (*a*) An oral iron preparation is usually adequate in infancy, e.g. ferrous sulphate BP 60 mg (0·2 mmol elemental iron) three times daily. Double these doses in toddlers (see p. 176).

(*b*) Parenteral iron is rarely necessary and is probably better avoided if the plasma transferrin concentration is low, e.g. in the newborn, the malnourished, or those with protein loss.

(*c*) Blood transfusion is occasionally necessary, e.g. if there is heart failure; frusemide should be given with the blood and 10 ml per kg of blood only should be infused over at least 6 hours (see p. 133).

(*d*) Source of blood loss (if any) should be treated; in some countries the most common cause is hookworm infestation (see p. 79).

Prevention: For preterm babies and twins 0·2 mmol elemental iron daily throughout infancy. Oral prophylactic iron should not be given if the baby is breast feeding to avoid saturating the lactoferrin.

Most formulae contain 0·02 mmol of elemental iron per 100 ml which is sufficient for normal babies.

Other iron-containing foods, e.g. iron-fortified cereals, green vegetables, egg, should be introduced between the 4th and 6th month of life.

COMMON PRIMARY NUTRITIONAL DISORDERS IN DEVELOPING COUNTRIES

Protein Energy Deficiency

Mild degrees of deficiency of energy and protein cause growth retardation; extreme degrees cause the syndromes of nutritional marasmus and kwashiorkor.

Treatment: Diet is the essential part of treatment but care is necessary with common complications such as hypothermia, hypoglycaemia, drowsiness, diarrhoea, heart failure, and infection. Using some of the foods shown in Table IV (p. 27) it is possible, using locally available products, to devise a diet which will provide 400–650 kJ (97–156 kcals), 2–4 g milk protein, 4–6 mmol potassium, 1–2 mmol magnesium and less than 3 mmol sodium per kg. body weight each day. A selection of milk-based diets are shown in Table IV. During the second week of treatment solids are added to the milk diet.

Prevention: For the individual family the aim is to achieve a good supply of protein foods by (*a*) encouraging prolonged breast feeding up to two years, (*b*) the use of locally available protein foods, e.g. ground-nuts, soya beans, etc., and (*c*) as a stop-gap the use of imported protein supplements such as dried skimmed milk from UNICEF.

Vitamin A Deficiency

Vitamin A deficiency is a major cause of blindness, particularly in the Middle East and South East Asia. Conjunctival keratosis and Bitot's spots occur, clouding of the cornea (xerosis) is a clinical emergency because it may go on to necrosis (keratomalacia) with scarring and sometimes perforation.

Treatment: Retinol (water miscible preparation) 3000 μg per kg body weight I.M. immediately.

3000 μg per kg body weight orally daily, days 2 to 6.

1500 μg daily thereafter until eyes are normal.

Associated kwashiorkor or marasmus should be treated at the same time.

Prophylaxis: Retinol (oily preparation) 300 µg daily by mouth, or 60,000 µg by mouth every 4 to 6 months (limited value only).

TABLE IV (*a*)
CASILAN DRIED SKIMMED MILK-SUCROSE DIET (CaDSu) FOR CHILDREN WITH KWASHIORKOR

Ingredients of the "dry" CaDSu diet		Nutritional value per 100 ml reconstituted diet	
Casilan	33 g	Protein	4·0 g
Dried skimmed milk	30 g	Fat	6·1 g
Sucrose	30 g	Carbohydrate	4·6 g
Cottonseed oil	60 g	Energy	375 kJ
Potassium chloride	2·7 g	Potassium	4·7 mmol
Magnesium chloride	0·3 g	Magnesium	0·7 mmol
		Sodium	0·9 mmol
Total	156 g		

The mixture of "dry" ingredients is prepared for use by taking 156 g of this mixture and making it into a paste with a little cold boiled water in scalded equipment, and then adding, gradually, enough cold sterile water to make a total of 1000 g. The reconstituted diet is fed at the rate of 100 ml per kg of body weight per day. Add Abidec 0·6 ml and folic acid 1 mg daily.

TABLE IV (*b*)
MILK-SUCROSE DIET (MSu) FOR CHILDREN WITH MARASMUS

Ingredients of the "dry" mixture		Nutritional value per 200 g of the reconstituted diet	
Full-cream milk powder	80 g	Protein	4·0 g
		Fat	14·3 g
Sucrose	35 g	Carbohydrate	13·2 g
Cottonseed oil	50 g	Energy	840 kJ
		Potassium	5·2 mmol
		Magnesium	0·8 mmol
Total	165 g	Sodium	2·8 mmol

The mixture of "dry" ingredients is prepared for use by taking 165 g of this mixture and mixing as for CaDSu in Table IV (*a*).

The reconstituted diet is fed at the rate of 200 g per kg body weight per day or to capacity.

Infantile Beriberi

This condition occurs in South East Asia in breast-fed infants of thiamine-deficient mothers who eat a polished rice diet.

In the cardiac form a diuresis within a few hours of giving parenteral thiamine hydrochloride—25 mg I.V. or 100 mg I.M.—is diagnostic as well as therapeutic. This emergency treatment is followed by 25 mg I.M. daily for three days, then 10 mg orally twice a day. The mother should be treated at the same time—10 mg orally twice a day. Treatment for other forms is the same.

Pellagra

Pellagra occurs in children usually of school age receiving a maize diet, particularly in South Africa. Evidence of general undernutrition is usually present, as well as the classical dermatitis on exposed areas.

Treatment should include nicotinamide orally 50 mg three times a day but a good mixed diet, including milk (to provide tryptophan) and supplements of the other B vitamins is necessary too. Very rarely intravenous nicotinamide 3 mg is necessary in the presence of severe anorexia and diarrhoea.

Prophylaxis: Diet should contain milk.

Iodine Deficiency

Goitres due to iodine deficiency may occur, particularly in adolescent girls, in many parts of the world; frank hypothyroidism is also occasionally present.

Treatment: Iodine 200 µg daily for 6 weeks, then 100 µg daily for prophylaxis.

DIETARY MANAGEMENT IN OTHER DISORDERS

Many transiently ill children require dietary attention and the diet may be an important aspect of the long-term treatment of many metabolic and gastro-intestinal disorders. This section gives details of diets in common use. A dietitian will be able to offer fuller and more varied regimes. *Diets for Sick Children* (1974), by D. E. M. Francis (Oxford: Blackwell Scientific), is useful for reference, and for proprietary preparations the manufacturer's data sheets should be consulted.

For many of the disorders dietary manipulation is only one aspect of management.

SPECIAL FORMULAE AND DIETS

Tables V to VIII give details of special formulae, food supplements, individual nutrients, and thickening agents in common use.

Table IX and the following pages give details of foods and special diets suitable for the older infant, toddler and school-child. Considerable skill is necessary to design, for children of this age, a diet which is therapeutically suitable and still attractive and palatable.

If a child's diet is very unusual, e.g. it is based on special formulae and/or isolated nutrients, then consideration of the quantity and quality of the nutritional intake is essential, i.e. the sources of nutrients (fluid, energy, protein, carbohydrate, fat), major minerals (sodium, potassium, magnesium, calcium, iron), vitamins (including the less commonly considered ones, e.g. inositol, biotin) and trace elements. It is often necessary to supplement such diets with vitamin and/or mineral mixtures (see p. 36).

Many of the formulae and foods detailed in the Tables are prescribable (see section on "Borderline Substances" in a current *MIMS*). EC10 forms should be headed "as per Clayton Committee".

Key to Abbreviations Used

Nutrient Source:

(*a*) Protein
    CM   Cow's milk (mainly casein)
    HC   Hydrolysed casein
    AA   Amino acids
    EAA   The eight essential acids for adults (i.e. no histidine or cysteine)

(*b*) Fat
    BF   Butter fat from cow's milk
    V   Vegetable derived (mainly poly-unsaturated long-chain)
    MCT Medium chain triglyceride, saturated fat

(c) Carbohydrate F   Fructose
                  G   Glucose
                  L   Lactose (glucose and galactose)
                  S   Sucrose (glucose and fructose)
                  HSt   Hydrolysate starch (glucose, mal-
                         tose and higher dextrins)
                  St   Starch

Manufacturers

A & H   Allen and Hanburys Limited, London, E2 6LA
Al   Alembic Prods., Oaklands House, Oaklands Drive,
        Sale, Manchester M33
B   Beecham Prods. Ltd., Gt. West Road, Brentford,
        Middx.
        Carlo Erba, 28–30 Great Peter Street, London SW1
        Carlosta, 33 Ermune Road, London SE13
C   Carnation Foods Ltd., Bush House, Aldwych,
        London WC2B 4QA
C & G   Cow and Gate Baby Foods, Guildford, Surrey GU1
D F   Duncan, Flockhart & Co. Ltd., Birkbeck Street,
        London E2
E   Eaton Laboratories, The Broadway, Woking, Surrey
        GU21 5AP
F   Fison Pharmaceuticals, Bakewell Road Lough-
        borough, Leics.
Ge   Geistlich Sons, Ltd., Newton Bank, Chester CH2 3QZ
Gl   Glaxo-Farley Foods Ltd., Plymouth, Devon PL3
M Jo   Mead Johnson, Stamford House, Langley, Slough,
        Berks SL3 6EB
N   Nestlé Co. Ltd., 36 Park Lane, Croydon, Surrey
        CR9 1NR
        Rite-Diet—Welfare Foods, 63–65 Higher Hillgate,
        Stockport, Cheshire
S H S   Scientific Hospital Supplies, 38 Queensland Street,
        Liverpool L7 3JG
        Sister Laura's Infant Food, Springfield Works,
        Bishopbriggs, Glasgow
Uni   Unigreg Ltd., 15–17 Worple Road, London SW19
W   Wander, 98 The Centre, Feltham, Middx. TW13 4EP

TABLE V

SUMMARY OF NUTRITIONAL PROPERTIES OF SPECIAL FEEDS
(Greater detail is given in Table VI)

Product	Protein		Carbohydrate		Fat			Others		
	Hydrolysed Casein or Non-Milk protein	Protein Content 15 g/l or less	Low Lactose/Galactose (traces only)	Sucrose/Fructose free	Low fat below 22 g/l	High proportion of Unsaturated Fats	Fat mainly as Medium Chain Triglycerides	Energy Content below 2·5 MJ (600 kcals) per litre	Low Sodium below 11 mmol/l	Vitamin and/or Mineral supplements required (see Table VI)
Albumaid Hydrolysate Complete	+		+*	+	+*			+	+	+
Allergilac				+				+		+
Comminuted Chicken	+		+*	+	+			+	+	+
Edosol				+		+			+	+
Flexical	+		+*			+	+			
Frailac		+			+			+	+	+
Galactomin 17			+	+		+		+	+	+
Galactomin 18			+	+	+	+		+	+	+
Galactomin 19			+		+	+		+	+	+
Locasol				+		+				+
LPLS		+		+		+			+	+
MCT (1) Milk			+			+	+**		+	+
Nutramigen	+		+*			+				
Portagen						+	+			
Pregestimil	+		+*			+	+			
Premium				+		+			+	
Prosol				+	+			+		+
SMA		+		+		+				
SMA Gold Cap		+		+		+			+	
Sobee/Prosobee	+		+			+				+
'V' Formula				+		+				
Velactin	+		+			+				+
Vivonex	+		+*	+	+	+				

* Completely Free
** Completely MCT Oil

Product		Allergilac (C & G)	Comminuted Chicken (C & G)	Edosol (C & G)	Frailac (C & G)	Galactomin 17 (C & G)	Galactomin 18 (C & G)	Galactomin 19 (C & G)	Locasol (C & G)	Lofenalac (M Jo)
Recommended Dilution w/v %		12½	50	12½	10	12½	12½	12½	12½	15
Protein g Source		34 CM	38 chicken	35 CM	12 CM	28 CM	28 CM	28 CM	27 CM	22[1]
Fat g Source		20 BF	13–20 chicken	35 V	12 V	28 V	18 V	18 V	29 V	27 V
Carbohydrate g Source		54 L	nil	47 L	72 77%S 23%L	63 HSt tr L	73 HSt tr L	73 F tr L	65 L	85 St HSt
	Na	59	2	2	8	6	6	6	10	26
Minerals	K	35	6·4	23	11	15	15	15	19	38
mmol	Ca	26	1	30	10	23	23	23	< 1·6	25
	P	28	7	27	10	19	19	19	16	23
Vitamins to be given [2] Mineral mixture required [2]		ADC	special YES	special YES	ADC	special YES	special YES	special YES	special yes but not Ca	
Energy Value/l MJ (kcals)		2·2 (520)	1·3 (300)	2·6 (630)	1·8 (420)	2·1 (500)	2·3 (540)	2·3 (550)	2·5 (600)	2·9 (700)

[1] Deficient in phenylalanine.
[2] See Table VIII.

VI

FEEDS—PER LITRE OF FEED

LPLS (C & G)	Minafen (C & G)	MCT (1) Milk (C & G)	Nutramigen (M Jo)	Portagen (M Jo)	Pregestimil (M Jo)	Prosol (C & G)	Sobee (M Jo)	Velactin (W)	Prososbee (M Jo)	Product
12½	15	12½	15	15	15	12½	15	15	1:1 in water	Recommended Dilution w/v %
10 CM	25¹	32 CM	23 HC	25 CM	21 HC	79 CM	33 Soya & Methionine	32 Soya & Methionine	26 Soya & Methionine	Protein g Source
32 V	62 V	35 MCT	27 V	34 87% MCT 13%V	27 75% MCT 25%V	1 BF	26 V	27 V	34 V	Fat g Source
78 ..%L 34% HSt	96 G HSt	51 HSt tr L	89 S St	80 HSt <1·6 gL	86 85%G 15% HSt	33 L	79 HSt S	74 G.Hst 2%S	68 G.Hst	Carbohydrate g Source
	28	5	14	19	18	65	22	10	18	
	16	16	18	27	24	22	41	9	19	Minerals
5	35	31	24	18	23	26	25	17	20	mmol
5	12	26	24	18	23	35	17	24	17	
ecial	special	special				ADC		ADC		Vitamins to be given²
ES		YES						YES		Mineral mixture required²
2·6 (630)	4·2 (1010)	2·6 (630)	2·9 (700)	2·9 (700)	2·8 (660)	1·9 (450)	2·9 (700)	2·8 (660)	2·8 (660)	Energy Value/l MJ (kcals)

TABLE VII

COMPOSITION OF DIETARY SUPPLEMENTS, LIQUID FEEDS, ETC. PER KG OF FOOD

Product, Manufacturer and recommended dilution (%) if any	PROTEIN SUPPLEMENTS						CARBOHYDRATE SUPPLEMENTS					
	Casilan (Gl)	Dried Skimmed Milk Powder (Domestic)	Forceval (Uni)	Aminonutrin (Ge)	Nefranutrin (Ge)	Albumaid Hydrolysate Complete (SHS)	Gastro Caloreen (SHS)	Caloreen (SHS)	Calonutrin (Ge)	Hycal (Liquid) (B)	Sucrose (Table sugar)	Glucodin (Gl)
Protein g / Source	900 CM	345 CM	550 CM	1000 AA	314 EAA	894* AA	0	0	0	0	0	0
Fat g / Source	18 BF	3 BF	10 BF	0	0	0	0	0	0	0	0	0
Carbohydrate g / Source	0	490 L	300 L	0	642 GSF	0	1000 HSt**	1000 HSt**	1000 HSt	610 HSt**	1000 S	1000 G
Minerals mmol — Na	4	260	<53	0	66	4	52	10	40	6	0.2	0
Minerals mmol — K	tr	342	13	0	4	0.5	1	1	3	2	0.6	0
Minerals mmol — Ca	298	317	345	0	0	0.7	0	0	0	6	0.3	0
Minerals mmol — P	258	364	65	0	0	1	0	0	0	0.7	tr	—
Energy MJ (kcal)	16.2 (3860)	13.7 (3260)	15.4 (3670)	16.8 (4000)	14.3 (3415)	15.0 (3576)	16.0 (4000)	16.8 (4000)	16.8 (4000)	10.2 (2440)	16.8 (4000)	16.8 (4000)

* This value has been corrected for moisture content.
** Predominance of higher sugars resulting in a low osmolarity.

Product, Manufacturer and recommended dilution (%) if any	FAT SUPPLEMENTS					LIQUID FEEDS			Elemental Diets (Use in young patients not yet fully established)		THICKENING AGENTS				
	M C T oil (Al, C & G, M Jo, SHS)	Cream (Single) (Domestic)	Cream (Double) (Domestic)	Prosparol (DF)	Corn Oil (Domestic)	Carnation Instant breakfast food*** (C) 16%	Complan**** (GI) 15-20%	Slender*** (C) 16%	Flexical*** (M Jo) 23%	Vivonex**** (E) 26.6%	Arrowroot (Domestic) 2-4%	Cornflour (Domestic) 2-4%	Bengers (F) 4%	Sister Laura's 2-7%	Carobel (C & G) 0.5-1% Nestargel (N) — Nutrients not available for absorption
Protein g Source	0	24·0 CM	15·0 CM	0	tr	23 C	200 CM	340 CM	99 HC	122 AA	4	5	100 Wheat	144 Wheat	
Fat g Source	999 MCT	212 BF	482 BF	500 V	999 V	5 B	160 V	8 BF	150 MCT & V	5 V	1	7	12	11	
Carbohydrate g Source	0	32 L	20 L	0	0	6-8 S & L	546 LS & HSt	572 S & L	678 S & HSt	863 G & HSt	940 St	920 St	830 St	820 St	
Minerals mmol — Na	0	18	12	0·7	tr	112	152	268	66	144	2	23	130		
K	0	32	20	0	tr	257	218	214	141	112	5	16	36		
Ca	0	19	13	0	tr	25	183	261	66	42	2	4	4		
P	0	14	7	0	tr	206	187	281	71	54	9	13	35		
Energy MJ (kcal)	34·8 (8300)	9·2 (2190)	19·4 (4620)	18·9 (4500)	39·0 (9300)	4·4 (4440)	18·5 (4440)	15·1 (3580)	18·5 (4400)	13·7 (3350)	15 (3550)	14·8 (3540)	16·0 (3800)	15·8 (3751)	

*** not chocolate flavour
**** plain vanilla or unflavoured

TABLE VIII
SOME AVAILABLE VITAMIN AND MINERAL SUPPLEMENTS

Preparation	Daily Recommended Dose	Vitamins A µg	B mg Thiamine	B mg Riboflavin	B mg Nicotinamide	B mg Pyridoxine	C mg	D µg	Vitamins Others	Minerals Sodium mmol	Potassium mmol	Magnesium mmol	Calcium mmol	Phosphorus mmol	Iron mmol	Minerals Others
ADC Vitamin mixtures DHSS Vitamin drops	7 drops but see p. 00	300	—	—	—	—	30	10	—	—	—	—	—	—	—	—
ABIDEC* (Parke Davis)	0·6 ml (0·3 ml in infancy)	1200	1·0	0·4	5·0	0·5	50	10	—	—	—	—	—	—	—	—
Adexoline Liquid (Glaxo)	0·4 ml	420	—	—	—	—	42	14	—	—	—	—	—	—	—	—
Special Vitamin mixtures Cow & Gate* Vitamin Tablets	12 tablets	—	3·0	3·0	10·0	1·0	120	—	E, K, B₁₂ Pantothenate Folic Acid, Biotin	tr	—	—	—	—	0·2	Zn, Mn, Cu, Mb, I
Ketovite syrup	5 ml syrup	940	—	—	—	—	—	10		—	—	—	—	—	—	—
plus Tablets (Paines & Byrne)	3 tablets	—	3·0	3·0	9·9	0·99	50	—	E, K, B₁₂ Pantothenate Folic Acid Biotin, Choline, Inositol	—	—	—	—	—	—	—
Aminogran Mineral Mixture (A & H)	1·5 g/kg up to maximum of 8 g	—	—	—	—	—	—	—	—	1·7	2·1	0·4	2·1	1·9	0·01	Cu, Zn, Mn I, Al, Co, Mb
Metabolic Mineral Mixture (SHS)	1·5 g/kg up to maximum of 8 g	—	—	—	—	—	—	—	—	1·7	2·1	0·4	2·1	1·9	0·01	Cu, Zn, Mn I, Al, Co, Mb

content per g of powder

TABLE IX

Summary of Nutritional Properties of Special Foods for Older Children

Product	gluten free	lactose/ milk free	Sucrose/ fructose free	Low protein < 0·5 g%	Low sodium < 0·3 mmol %
Carlo Erba:					
Aproten crispbread	+*			+*	
Pasta (various)	+*			+*	
Aproten flour	+*	+	+	+*	+
Carlosta:					
Azeta Biscuits (various)				+*	+
Pasta (various)				+*	+
Cow & Gate:					
Liga Biscuits					
Glutenex	+*	+			
Aminex		+*	+*	+*	+*
Glaxo-Farley:					
Farley Rusk		+			+
Farley Baby Rice with Egg	+				
Gluten-free Biscuit	+*				
Rite-Diet:					
Gluten-free Biscuits (various)	+*				
Gluten-free Bread-mix	+*				
Gluten-free cake	+				
Gluten-free flour	+*				
Low-protein bread	+*	+*	+*	+*	+
Low-protein flour	+*	+*	+*	+*	+
Robinson's:					
Baby Rice	+	+	+	+	+
Energen:					
Nutregen wheat starch flour	+*	+	+	+*	+

* These products are prescribable on EC10 for appropriate disorders.
Manufacturers of foods for infants and toddlers provide up-to-date lists of their gluten-free, milk-free, disaccharide-free, etc. products.

GLUTEN-FREE DIET FOR COELIAC DISEASE

In a gluten-free diet, all foods containing wheat and rye must be eliminated unless they have been specially treated to remove the gluten. It is best to avoid oats and barley too.

Foods allowed	**Foods forbidden**
Milk, cream, cheese, yoghurt.	Cheese spreads.
All meats and fish.	Sausages, meat and fish coated
Eggs, all fruits and vege-	with flour or breadcrumbs.
tables.	Tinned meat. Meat and fish
Butter, margarine vegetable	pasties.
oils, dripping, lard and cream.	Porridge. Breakfast cereals
Rice, tapioca, sago, cornflour	made from wheat or oats,
and custard powders.	e.g. Weetabix, Shredded
Breakfast cereals made from	Wheat, etc.
corn or rice, e.g. corn-	Semolina, spaghetti, mac-
flakes, Rice Krispies, gluten-	aroni and other pasta.
free bread, e.g. Rite-Diet.	Ordinary bread, cakes and
Sugar, honey, jam,	biscuits, flavoured crisps.
marmalade.	Malted bed-time drinks, e.g.
Tea, coffee, cocoa.	Horlicks.
Special products (see p. 37).	Certain chocolates, sweets
	and ice creams.

See p. 37 for details of gluten-free foods available on EC10. The Coeliac Society regularly publishes lists of gluten-free foods (P.O. Box 181, London NW2 2QY).

MINIMAL GALACTOSE AND LACTOSE DIET

Lactose is the disaccharide (glucose and galactose) found in milk and hence in all products made from or with milk. The minimal galactose diet shown is adequate for galacto-saemia, but occasionally even stricter limitation is necessary. Low-lactose diets are sometimes beneficial in gastro-intestinal disease and on occasion it may also be beneficial to limit the amount of sucrose, long-chain fat and gluten too. If special milk substitutes are used, a vitamin supplement may be required (see p. 36). An extended list of foods may be requested from a dietetic department.

Foods allowed	**Foods forbidden**
Prescribed Milk Substitute (see p. 31).	Milk, cream, butter, dried milk powders, cheese, yoghurt
CoffeeMate* (for older children).	ice cream.
Casilan.*	All tinned or prepared meats and fish or fish fingers.
Manufactured infant and toddler foods which *do not* include milk, milk solids, whey, cheese, lactose or monosodium glutamate. Check with manufacturers' lists and labels carefully.	Sausages. Milk and fancy breads. All baby cereals with milk solids, e.g. Farex. Coco Krispies, Special K, Alpen-type cereals. All other margarines.
Freshly cooked plain meats and fish.	All tinned milk puddings and tinned spaghetti with cheese.
Eggs.	Fudge, toffee, chocolate,
All fresh vegetables and fruit.	crisps.
Baked beans except with sausage.	Complan, Carnation Instant Breakfast Food.
All bread, except milk and fancy breads. Farley's Rusks, Robinson's Baby Rice, Cow & Gate (Liga) Glutenex Rusk. Cornflakes, Rice Krispies, Weetabix. Tomor margarine Outline spread, vegetable oils.	*All* drinking chocolate and malted milk powders A large variety of manu- factured foods contain skimmed milk and are un- suitable—check manufacturers' lists.
Dry cereals and pastas cooked in water or with milk sub- stitute. Jelly, boiled sweets, ice lollies (without ice cream/ toffee centres), pastilles, gums jam, syrup, sugar.	
Squash, fizzy pop, Oxo, Mar- mite and Bovril.	
Tea and coffee.	

*Contains milk-protein.

Low-sodium and Low-protein/High-protein Diets

These diets may be necessary in renal or liver disease. Sometimes potassium restriction is necessary too.

In Infancy

By choosing suitable formulae and supplements from Tables II, VI and VII it is possible to meet a variety of intakes, e.g.

Constituents	Low sodium below 8 mmol/l	Very low sodium* below 3 mmol/l
Low protein: below 1·2 g/l		LPLS
Normal protein: 1·5–2·0 g/l	Breast milk Gold Cap SMA	LPLS + Casilan
Moderate protein: 2·0–3·5 g/l	Gold Cap SMA + Casilan	Edosol
High protein: more than 3·5 g/l		Edosol + Casilan

*Caution is necessary with these very low sodium intakes.
Add baby rice (mixed with water) and/or special biscuits (see Table IX) after weaning.

Older Child

Food supplements from Table VII (p. 34) may be useful additions to the child's self-selected meagre diet particularly for short-term use and when dietetic advice is not immediately available, e.g. "High-energy, low-protein, sodium, potassium": Caloreen, Hycal, Prosparol, etc. "High-protein, low-sodium": Casilan, Forceval, Aminonutrin, etc. Note that doorstep milk and skimmed milk contain large amounts of sodium and potassium relative to their protein and energy content.

For longer-term management food tables and exchange lists must be consulted; a dietitian's help is invaluable. If possible energy intake should be maintained at 10 per cent over the normal intake for age, and protein intake should rarely be less than half the normal (see Table I). The children are often anorexic and food supplements are necessary to maintain growth. Liquid food supplements may be more acceptable to the anorexic child as a "medicine" morning and evening. This allows him a more free diet during the day (in effect restricted by his anorexia).

Low-Fat Diet (approximately 25 g)

This diet may be of value in malabsorption. When limiting dietary fat care is necessary to avoid also limiting associated nutrients, e.g. energy, protein, and fat-soluble vitamins. In malabsorption medium-chain triglyceride (MCT) oil or formula introduced slowly and/or carbohydrate supplements (see Tables V and VI) if they are tolerated, may be used as an energy supplement.

Diets used for the treatment of the hyperlipidaemias are commonly more restricted in long-chain fat than the one shown below; depending on the variety of the hyperlipidaemia, extra energy may be provided by polyunsaturated oils or MCT oil.

Foods allowed	**Foods forbidden**
Skimmed milk liquid or powder, Casilan.	Ordinary doorstep milk, cream, butter, margarine, cheese, ice cream.
White fish, lean meat either boiled, grilled or roast with no additional fat.	Eggs. All oils.
All fruit and vegetables.	All fatty meats (bacon, ham). Oily fish, canned meat and fish.
Clear vegetable soups.	
Robinson's Baby Rice.	Pastry, pies, sausages, gravy.
All adult breakfast cereals.	All fried foods.
Dried cereals and pasta cooked with water or milk substitute. Meringues.	Chips, fried vegetables. Cream soups.
Bread.	All cakes and biscuits. Doughnuts, fancy buns.
Jelly, water/plain ice lollies.	Chocolate, toffee, crisps, nuts, fudge.
Jam, honey, syrup, sugar, boiled sweets, sugar.	Lemon curd, peanut butter.
Fruit juice and squashes, fizzy pop, Bovril, Marmite, Oxo. Tea and coffee.	All chocolate and malted milk powders.

Additional portions of fat would be provided by:

1 egg (7 g), 5 g margarine or butter (4 g), 10 g Outline margarine (4 g).

B.A.W.
A.deL.

[NOTES]

[NOTES]

[NOTES]

III

FLUID AND ELECTROLYTE THERAPY

FLUID AND ELECTROLYTE THERAPY

Fluid and electrolyte therapy involves three basic considerations:

1. Provision of maintenance requirements.
2. Replacement of pre-existing deficits.
3. Correction of continuing losses.

MAINTENANCE REQUIREMENTS

Maintenance requirements of fluid and electrolytes are proportional to the child's calorie needs. Sick children may require more or less than usual, depending upon their metabolic rates. Persistent fever increases calorie and fluid requirements by 12 per cent for each degree centigrade rise.

MAINTENANCE I.V. FLUID AND ELECTROLYTE REQUIREMENTS

Body Weight	Calories/Day	Fluid ml/day	Sodium mmol/day	Potassium mmol/day
Less than 10 kg	100/kg	100–120/kg	2·5–3·5/kg	2·5–3·5/kg
10–20 kg	75–100/kg	90–120/kg	2·0–2·5/kg	2·0–2·5/kg
over 20 kg	45–75/kg	50–90/kg	1·5–2·0/kg	1·5–2·0/kg

Maintenance fluid and sodium requirements are most conveniently administered as 0·18 per cent sodium chloride and dextrose 4 per cent injection. The glucose supplied does not satisfy calorie needs but will prevent the development of ketosis, if oral feeding has been stopped. Note that intravenous fluid requirements are less than oral.

REPLACEMENT OF PRE-EXISTING DEFICIT

In practice, deficits are most easily expressed in terms of body weight.

Estimation of Dehydration—expressed as a percentage of body wt.

> mild—5%: decreased skin turgor;
> dry mucous membranes.

moderate—10%: increased severity of above signs;
sunken fontanelle;
reduced intra-ocular pressure;
tachycardia, oliguria.

severe—15%: marked increase in severity of above signs;
drowsiness, hypotension.

Types of dehydration.—Three types are recognised, resulting from variable loss of sodium in relation to water:

hypotonic – serum sodium < 130 mmol/l
isotonic   – serum sodium 130–150 mmol/l
hypertonic – serum sodium > 150 mmol/l.

The degree of dehydration may be underestimated in hypertonic states, due to increased cell turgor.

Calculation of Replacement in Hypotonic and Isotonic Dehydration

This requires a knowledge of the normal distribution of body fluids and electrolytes, the patient's electrolyte levels and blood H^+ concentration, and the electrolyte content of infusion solutions.

Fluid volume replacement (litres) = % dehydration × body wt in kg;

Sodium replacement (mmols) = (140—serum Na mmol/l) × total body water.

The total body water is 75 per cent of body weight up to 1 month, 70 per cent up to 1 year and 65 per cent up to 12 years of age.

The serum sodium value should approximately equal chloride + bicarbonate values + 10 mmols/litre. Discrepancy suggests the presence of other anions in unusual concentrations, e.g. ketoacids or phosphate.

Potassium levels in serum are a poor guide to the state of total body potassium, particularly in the presence of dehydration, hyponatraemia and acidosis, which raises the serum potassium. It should be given orally unless precluded by vomiting, and should not be commenced until urine flow is established and the blood urea is falling to normal. It may be added to intravenous fluids in an amount of 3·0 mmol/kg/24 hrs, in a maximum concentration of 40 mmol/l. Too rapid administration can produce dangerously elevated serum levels. ECG monitoring is useful in severe cases.

Acidosis will correct spontaneously as the circulation and renal function improve, calories are given, and electrolyte loss subsides. Calculation of the bicarbonate needed to correct acidosis is not precise, while over-rapid and full correction may increase CSF acidosis. The amount of bicarbonate required

= base deficit (mmol/l) × body wt (kg) × 0·3 = mmol for full correction

Half this amount should be given over 24 hours. In severe acidosis (base deficit > 10 mmol/l) an initial 1 mmol/kg may be given well diluted in the replacement fluids over the first 2 hours.

Composition of solutions for intravenous use in mmol/l.

	Na^+	K^+	Cl^-
Sodium chloride injection (0·90%)	154	—	154
Sodium chloride (0·18%) and dextrose (4%) injection	30·8	—	30·8
Hartmann's	130	4	104
Citrated plasma	150	12	55

1 ml of 8·4% sodium bicarbonate contains

1 mmol bicarbonate;
1 mmol sodium

1 g of potassium chloride contains 13 mmol of potassium;
13 mmol of chloride

1 ml Inj. calcium gluconate B.P. 10% contains
0·225 mmol Ca^{++}

1 ml Inj. calcium chloride B.P. $CaCl_2.2H_2O$ contains
0·5 mmol Ca^{++}

Calculation of millimoles

One millimole = molecular weight in milligrams.
Useful atomic wts:

hydrogen	1·0	magnesium	24·3
carbon	12·0	phosphorus	31·0
nitrogen	14·0	chlorine	35·5
oxygen	16·0	potassium	39·1
sodium	23·0	calcium	40·1

therefore, for example:

1 mmol NaCl = 58·5 mg. 1 mmol NaHCO$_3$ = 84 mg.
1 mmol KCI = 74·6 mg. 1 mmol NH$_4$Cl = 53·5 mg.

CORRECTION OF CONTINUING LOSSES

These losses are usually from the gastro-intestinal or renal tract. Replacement should be contemporaneous, the fluids being of similar composition to those lost, their volume being calculated every 6–8 hours. In small infants with large continuing losses waiting for a 24-hr period to calculate replacement is too long.

Electrolyte composition of alimentary fluids (mmol/l)

	H +	Na$^+$	K$^+$	Cl$^-$	HCO$_3^-$
Gastric	40–60	20–80	5–20	100–150	—
Small Bowel	—	100–140	5–15	90–130	20–40
Biliary	—	120–140	5–15	80–120	30–50
Diarrhoea	—	40	40	40	40
(stool water, mean)					

In sodium depletion due to renal loss the urinary sodium concentration is high (> 40 mmol/l), when unrelated to renal disease urinary sodium concentration is extremely low (< 10 mmol/l).

Practical Management of Hypotonic or Isotonic Dehydration

1. *If the patient is more than 5 per cent dehydrated or is shocked.*

   Give isotonic solution, such as 0·9 per cent saline, or plasma at 20 ml/kg over 2 hrs, then continue as 2.

2. *If the patient is less than 5 per cent dehydrated.*

   (a) For maintenance give 0·18 per cent saline in 4 per cent dextrose as per table on page 51.

   (b) Replace three-quarters of the dehydration deficit as calculated on page 48 as 0·18 per cent saline or 0·9 per cent saline according to the degree of hyponatraemia. Aim to correct half the bicarbonate deficit and also add potassium chloride (3 mmol/kg/24 hrs) after urine flow is established and the blood urea is falling towards normal.

3. Monitor serum electrolytes, osmolality and H^+ concentration on admission and after 2, 12, and 24 hours. Record fluid intake and output accurately, and weigh the patient daily.

I.V. fluids given to infants should be administered in a graduated chamber or divided into four equal portions in order to prevent inadvertent sudden fluid overload.

ROUGH GUIDE TO REHYDRATION

(First 24 hours, excluding newborn)

Basic fluid will be 0·18 per cent saline in 4 per cent dextrose.

Weight kg	5% dehydration At 150 ml/kg/24 hr		10% dehydration Initial infusion of 0·9% saline or plasma in 2 hours then 200 ml/kg/24 hr	
	ml/24 hr	ml/hr	ml/24 hr	ml/hr
2	300	12	400*	17*
3	450	19	600*	25*
4	600	25	800*	33*
5	750	31	1000*	42*
6	950	40	1200*	50*
7	1050	44	1400*	58*
8	1200	50	1600*	67*
9	1350	56	1800*	75*
10	1500	63	2000*	83*

For additions of bicarbonate or potassium and adjustment of sodium intake, see text.

* If infant hypernatraemic give half to two-thirds this volume and rate, see text.

Hypernatraemic Dehydration

Intracellular fluid loss predominates initially so that the classical features of dehydration and circulatory failure develop slowly. The skin is of a doughy consistency and neurological features may be prominent. Most cases result from loss of hypotonic fluid, i.e. greater water than electrolyte loss; however some may result from excess sodium administration. Gradual reduction of the serum sodium over 2–3 days is essential to avoid CNS disturbance. Hypocalcaemia may be present and should be corrected.

Fluid administration.—1. Despite appearances many infants require initial repletion of the circulating blood volume using plasma or 0·9 per cent saline, 20 ml/kg over 1–2 hours.

2. Maintenance solutions thereafter should be hypotonic, preferably 0·18 per cent saline in 4 per cent dextrose at a rate no faster than 100 ml/kg/24 hour.

Potassium and bicarbonate supplements and patient monitoring are carried out as detailed above.

If oliguria persists or hypernatraemia has resulted from excess sodium chloride administration, peritoneal dialysis may be required.

Metabolic Alkalosis

This may occur following persistent vomiting as in pyloric stenosis, in cases of potassium loss and sodium retention, and following the administration of excess alkali. It is usually a self-correcting condition if renal function is good and the precipitating cause eliminated. If alkalosis is severe and tetany is imminent, it may be necessary to give anion with a readily disposable cation, e.g. ammonium chloride. The amount used is:

mmol chloride = base excess (HCO_3^-) mmol/l × 0·3 × body wt kg.

During a period of alkalosis excess potassium is lost in the urine. Extreme degrees of non-respiratory alkalosis may prove resistant to therapy until any potassium deficit is corrected.

Blood

The infant's blood volume is 8 per cent (80ml/kg) of the body weight, so that a transfusion of 20 ml/kg will raise the haemoglobin by approximately 25 per cent.

Parenteral Nutrition

This should be considered in any infant whose nutritional intake is inadequate for prolonged periods (e.g. more than one week), and consists of the intravenous administration of amino acids, carbohydrates, fat, minerals, trace elements and vitamins. It may be total or partial as a supplement to an insufficient oral intake.

Parenteral nutrition may be administered through peripheral or central veins. The peripheral route avoids the major risks of infection in a central venous cannula and is a simpler procedure; however the maximum daily calorie intake possible is quite limited, and drip sites may not be available. Sterile solutions should be prepared in a pharmacy, to contain vamin, glucose, electrolytes and vitamins. Fat is given as intralipid, trace minerals are given in plasma, and vitamin K, B_{12}, folic acid and iron are administered intramuscularly on a weekly basis.

If intravenous nutrition is required for more than three weeks, the central route is preferred. In view of the dangers of metabolic disturbance and infection which may arise, such patients should be managed in units experienced in the techniques involved.

M.J.B.

[NOTES]

[NOTES]

[NOTES]

IV

THE NEWBORN

GENERAL CARE AT BIRTH

THE following information should be obtained by telephone from the midwife, doctor or hospital. Accurate estimation of gestation. Bleeding or toxaemia. Maternal blood groups and antibodies. Membrane rupture to delivery interval. Mechanical factors at delivery. Fetal distress. Resuscitation response. Drugs used in labour with times of administration. Also required is history of previous births, stillbirths, neonatal disease and chronic disease in the family.

Infant Resuscitation

Equipment needed:
Mucus catheter. Funnel. Nasal catheter.
Infant face-mask and bag.
Endotracheal tubes, 2 of each (Warne's 8, 10, 12, 14, F.G.).
Suction catheters, 3 (Portsmouth pattern size 5).
Laryngoscope with infant blade and spare bulb and batteries.
Endotracheal connectors (Magill) 0, 00.
Infant Guedel portex airways 0, 00, 000.
1 or 2 ml syringes 2.
Ampoules of levallorphan.
Scissors, tape, oxygen source, reducing valve and flow-meter.

At birth note the time and gently clear mouth and nose. Dry carefully to reduce heat loss and wrap in warm blanket. Record Apgar scores at 1 and 5 minutes. Stimulate, by firmly slapping the soles of the feet and when the infant gasps support inspiration with face-mask and bag. If there is no response aspirate and intubate under direct vision; in the presence of meconium soiling of larynx, suck out through an endotracheal tube before applying positive pressure. This should be given with O_2 at maximum inflation pressure 30 cm of water by short inspiratory puffs 30–60/min sufficient to cause the chest wall to rise. Use levallorphan 0·25 mg (0·25 ml solution) I.M. or I.V. if the mother has recently received pethidine or morphia.*

If the heart is not beating, intubate and give cardiac massage by pressure with two fingers over middle-third of sternum

---

*Naloxone Neonatal now commercially available—*see* manufacturer's literature.

depressing it by about 1 cm at a rate of 100–200/min. The rhythm should be 8 chest compressions to 3 inflations with O_2 until spontaneous heart action is maintained. If infant is still limp and poorly responsive after I.P.P.R., sodium bicarbonate should be given via umbilical vein in a dose of 5 to 10 mmol according to size. Persistent or recurrent apnoea is usually caused by cerebral depression. Diaphragmatic hernia, pneumothorax, choanal atresia and hydrothorax need consideration. Prognosis is very poor if cardiac arrest > 5 min.

Note: maternal drugs including diazepam and chlormethiazole ("Heminevrin") may produce prolonged hypotonia and apnoea.

Phytomenadione 0·5 mg should be given to all infants below 2·5 kg and to those with complicated deliveries.

EXAMINATION OF THE NEWBORN

The first examination should be made shortly after birth. The aim is to assess the infant's general condition and his respiratory function, to find any treatable congenital malformation and to determine whether any special management is required in the first few days. A second examination should also be carried out at 7 to 10 days to assess weight gain, to exclude infection and to note significant cardiac murmurs.

AT BIRTH

1. Is the infant breathing easily?
2. Is the general appearance and skin colour satisfactory and muscle tone and posture normal?
3. If weight under 2·5 kg is the infant premature or small for dates or both?
4. Is a generalised disorder such as Down's syndrome present?
5. Search for malformations e.g. cleft palate, cataract, imperforate anus, sexual ambiguity and unstable hips. Oesophageal atresia should be excluded if there was hydramnios (see p. 69). 5 per cent of those with single umbilical artery have associated malformation.

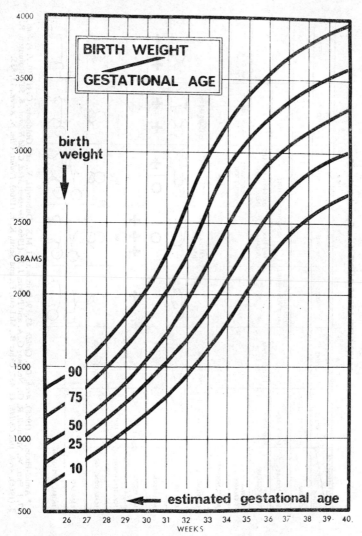

FIG. 1.—Intra-uterine weight chart. (After Lubchenko, L. D., Hansman C., Dressler, M., and Boyd, E. (1963). *Pediatrics*, **32,** 793–800.)

MATURITY ASSESSMENT (from Several Authors)*

GESTATION AGE / SIGNS	28 WEEKS	30 WEEKS	32 WEEKS	34 WEEKS	36 WEEKS	38 WEEKS	40 WEEKS
OEDEMA	HANDS, FEET, TIBIA				NONE		
SKIN TEXTURE	VERY THIN VEINS EASILY SEEN	THIN AND SMOOTH LARGE VEINS VISIBLE		VEINS HARDLY VISIBLE			
SKIN COLOUR	DARK RED	UNIFORM PINK		PALE PINK VARIABLE	PALE PINK EARS, LIPS, PALMS, SOLES		
PLANTAR SKIN CREASES					MAJOR CREASES FORE 1/3 SOLE	MAJOR CREASES 2/3 SOLE	MAJOR AND MINOR CREASING
BREAST NODULE					2 mm	4 mm	7 mm
EAR FIRMNESS		NO RECOIL		CARTILAGE SOFT IN PLACES		INSTANT RECOIL	
POSTURE							
ARM RECOIL				O	O +	+ +	+ +
LEG RECOIL			+	+ +	+	+ +	+ +
POPLITEAL ANGLE	150°		110°	100°	100°	90°	
SCARF SIGN		NO RESISTANCE					
HEAD LAG							
VENTRAL SUSPENSION							

* Amiel-Fison, C. (1968). Arch. Dis. Childh. 43, 89. Dubowitz, L.M.S., Dubowitz, V., and Goldberg, C. (1970). J. Pediat., 77, 1. Farr, V., Mitchell, R. G., Neligan, G. A. and Parkin, J. M. (1966). Develop. Med. Child Neurol., 8, 507. Robinson, R. J. (1966). Arch. Dis. Childh. 41, 437. Usher R., McLean, F., and Scott, K. E. (1966). Pediat. Clin. N. Amer., 13, 835.

SECOND EXAMINATION—AT 7–10 DAYS

1. Is the baby feeding well and gaining weight?—if not exclude infection and if negative think of cystic fibrosis, renal insufficiency, adrenal hyperplasia.
2. Look for infection on the skin, nails, eyes, mouth and umbilicus.
3. Does jaundice persist?
4. Is oedema present?
5. Are the liver, spleen, kidneys and heart normal? Are the hips stable?

SPECIAL PROBLEMS

Hypothermia

Common after delivery. Incubator or other external heat source such as electric cot pads (max. temp. 37·5°C), or overhead radiant heaters, help to restore temperature.

Low Birth Weight Babies

Temperature control.—Maintain the rectal temperature at 37°C. Small infants may need clothing or a plastic heat shield in the incubator to reduce radiant loss.

Feeding.—Early feeding is recommended to help in preventing hypoglycaemia, hyperbilirubinaemia and possibly other causes of brain damage. Start feeding at two hours if possible, using EBM or reconstituted infant formula. Earlier positive calorie/protein balance may be achieved by continuous duodenal/jejunal feeding through appropriate indwelling tube.

Standard regime: 1st day 45 ml/kg birth weight; 2nd day 60 ml/kg; 3rd day 80 ml/kg; 4th day 105 ml/kg. Daily increments are then added so that the intake reaches 200 ml/kg at two weeks.

Frail or ill infants may only be able to tolerate small feeds in the first few days until bowel function is established. Intravenous feeding may be required to prevent dehydration if feeds are not tolerated. Use 5 per cent dextrose 60–70 ml/kg/day for 48 hours, then 0·18 per cent saline in 4 per cent dextrose in increasing amounts to 110 ml/kg/day. Calcium and potassium supplements may be required [potassium 2 mmol/kg/day and approximately 5–10 ml calcium gluconate (10 per cent) per 100 ml infusate].

Vitamin supplements (see page 20) can be given from the age of one month and iron (see page 25) even earlier if indicated. The latter will need to be continued for the first 9–12 months of life.

Oxygen.—An ambient (incubator) concentration of over 40 per cent oxygen is dangerous unless the baby is cyanosed. The minimum level needed to overcome cyanosis may be checked by keeping the radial artery PaO_2 below 21 kPa (160 mmHg) or the umbilical artery levels between 8 kPa (60 mmHg) and 12 kPa (90 mmHg) to allow for the effect of a ductal shunt. Use local anaesthetic before radial artery puncture.

Light for Dates Baby

The weight is less than that on the 10th centile for gestation on the Lubchenko intra-uterine growth chart (see page 61.) Dry cracked skin, meconium staining, absence of body fat, disproportionate length or head size for weight all suggest the diagnosis. The gestation may be estimated from the E.D.D. by clinical measurement and neurological assessment (see chart). The main problems are hypoxia at birth and hypoglycaemia in next 48 hours.

Action

(a) 6-hourly Dextrostix for 48 hours. See p. 65 for treatment of hypoglycaemia.

(b) Feeding.—Larger feeds are needed to offset the hypoglycaemia which most commonly appears in the first 48 hours. The feed volume should be appropriate for a baby on the 25th centile for the estimated gestation. The baby usually feeds hungrily and gains weight without an initial loss. If I.V. feeding is necessary use low birth weight schedule (p. 63) after estimating what the weight would be for the 25th centile. Daily plasma electrolyte estimations are needed.

Infant of Diabetic Mother

Unless there is rigid maternal diabetic control complications may be expected. Delivery is usually induced around the 37th week of gestation. The behaviour is very immature in spite of deceptive macrosomia, plethora and Cushingoid appearance. Polycythaemia is usual and early hypocalcaemia common.

Action

(a) Apnoea monitor in incubator.

(b) Dextrostix at 2 hours then 6-hourly;

If blood glucose is: < 25 mg/100 (1·5 mmol/l) in first 12 hours
< 20 mg/100 (1 mmol/l) at 12–24 hours

treat with 10 per cent dextrose through umbilical vein catheter. If higher concentrations are needed peripheral veins must be used. Glucagon I.M. may be effective.

(c) Feeds.—6 one-hourly feeds of 10–15 ml of 10 per cent dextrose, EBM or Infant Formula, then according to standard feed regime.

MAJOR SYMPTOMS IN THE NEWBORN

RESPIRATORY DISTRESS

The causes may be placed into four approximately equal numerical groups thus:

1. **Gross pulmonary lesions.**—Massive aspiration and pneumonia are the most common. Pneumothorax is often not diagnosed. Cysts and lobar emphysema are rare. Diagnosis is made by careful examination followed by radiography. Remember to check membrane rupture/delivery interval and consider whether instrumentation could have introduced infection.

2. **Idiopathic respiratory distress syndrome** (I.R.D.S.) of the preterm infant presents from or shortly after birth and gradually worsens over the first few hours with chest retraction and grunting. Early X-ray excludes other conditions, but I.R.D.S. changes may be minimal. The difficulty in excluding pneumonia necessitates the use of antibiotic in some cases (see page 73).

3. **Cardiac conditions.**—Usually due to acyanotic lesions presenting with heart failure after 24 to 48 hours. Grunting is unusual but some cyanosis may be present. Liver enlarges. Cyanotic heart lesions usually present from birth with cyanosis but little distress, and often without relief in 100 per cent oxygen. For diagnosis and treatment see page 103.

4. **Extrapulmonary causes.**—The most common is cerebral trauma; other important causes include oesophageal atresia (see page 69), diaphragmatic hernia, choanal atresia, vascular rings and micrognathia. (Methaemoglobinaemia should not

be forgotten if cyanosis is present without respiratory changes).

Treatment in the absence of a remediable cause listed above remains symptomatic. The airway is kept clear by repeated aspiration, O_2 given for cyanosis and antibiotics when infection suspected or cannot be excluded. If nasal obstruction is present use oral airway held in by tapes attached to tube gauze helmet.

Essential Measures in R.D.S.

If breathlessness appears within a few hours of birth check temperature and if low restore to 37°C. If symptoms persist check Astrup values, pass gastric or duodeno-jejunal tube and start small frequent or continuous feeds; X-ray check to exclude other lesions and insert an umbilical catheter. If facilities for measuring arterial oxygen are available an umbilical arterial catheter can be used for administering parenteral fluids and obtaining specimens. Correct metabolic acidosis (p. 49) and if functional bowel ileus is present supply all fluids parenterally.

Oxygen is given to overcome cyanosis preferably monitored on arterial specimens (p. 137). If baby requires more than 50 per cent inspired oxygen to maintain umbilical arterial oxygen above 7 kPa (50 mmHg) consider use of C.P.A.P.

Warnings: 1. Babies with R.D.S. do not tolerate handling.
2. Aspiration of oral feeds is a constant problem.
3. The arterial oxygen may suddenly rise in the recovery phase.
4. Record how much blood is taken from the baby. Replacement transfusion may be required.

Antibiotics may be indicated not only for prophylaxis in case of inhalation of infected material but also because in some cases it is difficult to differentiate between neonatal pneumonia and idiopathic respiratory distress.

Apnoeic Attacks of the Immature

Periods of apnoea are common in very immature babies in the first few days but a late onset may follow the unsuspected aspiration of vomit or be the presenting symptom of some other major problem. Treatment consists of pharyngeal suction and oxygen. Intubation may be necessary. Use an apnoea monitor from birth in babies at risk. Repeated attacks may be overcome with continuous O_2 enrichment kept below 40 per cent unless infant is constantly cyanosed. Use of aminophylline suppositories 5 mg every 6 hours appears to be an effective deterrent and so does C.P.A.P. Assisted ventilation may be needed for repeated severe attacks.

Convulsions and other Cerebral Symptoms

Difficulties with ventilation, apnoea, alterations of tone, loss of suck and irritability may date from birth. A later onset of these symptoms, often preceded by lethargy or the presence of convulsions, oculogyric crises or a tense fontanelle demands the immediate exclusion of infection and biochemical disorders. Blood sugar and calcium, and/or lumbar puncture are urgently needed according to the clinical findings.

Intracranial Injury or Hypoxia

Lack of oxygen rather than frank mechanical injury is considered to be the main cause of brain damage at or around birth.

Symptoms usually arise within 48 hours of delivery and a history of fetal distress or difficulty in initiating respiration are common. The diagnosis may sometimes only be reached by excluding the treatable biochemical and infective states. It may present as hypoglycaemia with disappointing clinical response to treatment.

Neonatal Meningitis

Unexplained illness, unstable temperature, convulsion, apnoeic attack, prolonged jaundice may be the sole indication for immediate lumbar puncture. History of maternal illness, complicated delivery or low birth weight increases suspicion. Blood culture, throat swab, umbilical swab may yield suspected organism if CSF does not. The usual organisms are *E. coli*, proteus, streptococci or staphylococci. Salmonella, listeria and pneumococcus are less common. Infective organism may also be found in maternal high vaginal swab. Treatment will consist of chloramphenicol, penicillin, kanamycin, gentamicin, streptomycin, or sulphonamides, singly or in combination.

Hypoglycaemia

Irritability, twitching, fits, lethargy or irregular respirations may be symptoms and the baby is often small for dates. Early feeding may prevent this dangerous condition.

If the Dextrostix is non-recording take blood for glucose and treat if it is below 1 mmol/l (20 mg/100 ml). Use dextrose 10 or 20 per cent (10 per cent being the maximum permissible via the umbilical vein) in dose of 1 g/kg and continue oral feeds hourly. If blood glucose remains low give dextrose continuously I.V. and if this also fails prednisone 0·5 mg/kg 8-hourly or ACTH 5 units may be given.

Hypocalcaemia

Neonatal tetany is usually restricted to babies fed full-cream dried cow's milk and occurs around the 7th day. It may occur earlier in the ill, the immature or the babies of diabetic mothers. The aetiology here is less clear. Fits may be focal and even isolated local muscle twitching may occur. Serum calcium is below 1·75 mmol/l (7 mg/100 ml) and the phosphorus above 2·2 mmol/l (7 mg/100 ml).

Treatment with calcium gluconate 30 mg/kg (0·3 ml/kg of 10 per cent solution diluted to 2·5 per cent with water) by slow intravenous injection should give a diagnostically rapid control of the fits. For several days afterwards give calcium chloride 33 mg/kg, or calcium lactate 75 mg/kg four times daily orally to prevent relapse. Calcium chloride may occasionally give rise to acidosis. (Note that the only commercially available liquid preparation is calcium gluconate Sandoz.) Change to low-phosphorus infant formula or EBM.

Hypomagnesaemia

Should be considered when hypocalcaemic fits do not respond to treatment, and other causes have been excluded. Phosphorus may be normal high or low. Emergency treatment consists of 0·15 mmol/kg (0·075 ml/kg 50 per cent injection magnesium sulphate) I.M. or I.V. slowly followed by magnesium chloride $MgCl_2.6H_2O$ 30 mg/kg orally 4 times a day until normal levels are achieved.

GASTRO-INTESTINAL SYMPTOMS

Oesophageal Atresia with Tracheo-oesophageal Fistula

This presents with excess frothing and cyanotic attacks. In the first few hours of life gaseous abdominal distension is common. Hydramnios is often a pointer. Early diagnosis is vital and can be made in most instances by passing a wide bore catheter through the mouth into the oesophagus. If the catheter's progress is arrested or loops back, atresia is likely. An X-ray will show that a radio-opaque catheter is coiled in the upper pouch. In suspected cases nothing should be given by mouth until the condition has been excluded.

Vomiting

In the first 24 to 48 hours vomiting may result from swallowed blood or liquor. Persistent vomiting, vomiting of green material, failure of the stools to "change" to brown from dark meconium after 3 days and abdominal distension all suggest the presence of intestinal obstruction. Plain X-ray films of the abdomen will be needed to differentiate between atresia of the duodenum or small intestine, meconium ileus, malrotation of gut and Hirschsprung's disease.

These gross organic conditions can be simulated clinically by central vomiting from cerebral irritation, hiatus hernia, rectal mucous plug, inspissated meconium or ganglion-blocking agents given to the mother. Vomiting may be secondary to infection while excessive weight loss and dehydration at the end of the first week suggest the salt-losing form of the adreno-genital syndrome, see page 95. At this age infantile pyloric stenosis may also begin to give symptoms.

An intravenous drip, cross-matched blood and vitamin K are pre-operative necessities.

Plethora and Polycythaemia

The viscosity of blood rises rapidly when venous PCV > 70 per cent. If neurological or respiratory symptoms are also present dilution exchange 20–30 ml/kg with plasma may be considered.

PALLOR, SHOCK, HAEMORRHAGE

Fetal blood loss into the mother or through the placental anastomoses into an identical twin may be gradual before birth or sudden at birth. The haemoglobin level may be normal after a recent bleed. A feto-maternal bleed is confirmed by a Kleihauer test on the mother's blood, taken as soon as possible after birth. Haemorrhagic shock may also follow bleeding into the leg muscles in breech delivery, haemorrhage from the cord or the placenta at birth, or from the umbilical stump and gut or viscus particularly during the 2nd, 3rd or 4th day. If the baby is shocked, treat with an immediate transfusion with O Rh–ve blood. Deficiency of clotting factors enhances tendency to bleed so give vitamin K_1 (phytomenadione) 1·0 mg I.M. which will correct prothrombin lack. For more rapid correction use 10 ml/kg of fresh frozen plasma. Bleeding into an abdominal organ usually gives rise to a palpable mass and later staining around the umbilicus; bleeding into the adrenal may give the additional alarming symptoms of acute adrenal insufficiency which will require intravenous hydrocortisone as well as blood, see page 96. Purpura and bleeding from disseminated intravascular coagulation may occur in the ill baby. Low platelet count, low fibrinogen and presence of fibrin degradation products confirms. Effective correction of primary condition is the only useful treatment at present, but see page 132.

Unexplained Jaundice

Serum bilirubin levels rise in all newborn babies for the first 3 days of life. In about 30 per cent the serum level exceeds 85 μmol/l (5 mg/100 ml) and jaundice becomes visible. Jaundice developing within 24 hours of birth, becoming deep or persisting more than 7 days needs investigation as to its cause and careful observation of its course.

The hyperbilirubinaemia may cause brain damage and need treatment as detailed under haemolytic disease in the next section. REMEMBER: Light breaks down bilirubin: protect blood samples with dark wrapping.

Clinical jaundice within 12 hours is nearly always due to haemolytic disease of the newborn. Compare maternal and infant ABO/Rh groups and do Coombs' test.

Prematurity is associated with a greater incidence and level of hyperbilirubinaemia.

Sepsis remains an important cause for unexplained icterus and should always be considered. Here bilirubin may be unconjugated, conjugated or both. Check urine, take blood culture and clotted blood for toxoplasmosis, CMV and rubella antibodies.

Other causes such as galactosaemia, hypothyroidism, hepatitis, and atresia of the bile ducts usually present later, the latter two with signs of obstruction to the outflow of bile.

G-6-PD deficiency is rare in the U.K. but is a common cause of jaundice in Mediterranean races, Chinese, but less so in Indians and Negroes.

Some drugs such as chloramphenicol, salicylates and steroids compete with the conjugating mechanism, others such as sulphonamides compete for albumin binding and some such as vitamin K increase haemolysis.

HAEMOLYTIC DISEASE AND JAUNDICE OF THE NEWBORN

Haemolytic disease should be suspected if the mother is rhesus negative with rhesus antibodies, or group O with immune anti-A or anti-B antibodies. Often however O-A and O-B incompatibility cannot be detected antenatally. At birth if the clinical condition of the baby is bad with pallor, oedema and enlargement of liver and spleen, a small exchange transfusion with fully packed cells is indicated to correct anaemia. Digitalisation with aspiration of fluid from pleura and peritoneum may be necessary in the infant with anaemic heart failure.

If the infant is not *in extremis* the results of the cord blood findings can be awaited. Note that heel prick samples give 3–4 g/dl higher haemoglobin results, especially if there is delay in taking sample. If the haemoglobin is below 10 g/dl (70 per cent) immediate exchange with fully packed cells is indicated. If the haemoglobin lies between 10 g/dl and 14 g/dl it is usually possible to watch the serum bilirubin levels and carry out an exchange to keep the indirect bilirubin below 340 μmol/l (20 mg/100 ml).

A rise of serum bilirubin of more than 8·5 μmol/l (0·5 mg/100 ml) per hour usually indicates that the rate of haemolysis is exceeding the excretory powers of the liver, i.e. higher than 200 μmol/l (12 mg/100 ml) at 24 hours.

Prematurity biases towards early exchange because of the less efficient conjugation by the premature baby's liver.

Cord bilirubin levels are of little help in assessing need for immediate exchange transfusion except that infants with a cord bilirubin over 85 μmol/l (5 mg/100 ml) nearly always come to exchange transfusions in the end. The Coombs' test merely indicates that the infant is affected by rhesus incompatibility and it may be negative in O-A or O-B haemolytic disease.

Management of Jaundice

Prevention.—Small doses of phenobarbitone to the mother for three days before delivery in preterm or rhesus problems may stimulate hepatic enzymes.

Treatment.—Phototherapy slows the rate of rise of bilirubin and will usually control non-haemolytic jaundice, but with steeply rising levels or those exceeding 250 mol/l (15 mg/100 ml) *always* cross-match and reserve compatible blood for immediate exchange.

Exchange Transfusion

Blood should be obtained from both the baby and from the mother because it is essential to make sure that the donor cells and the maternal serum are compatible. Compatible Rh–ve blood should always be used in rhesus disease and packed if the infant is anaemic; whole blood should be used for babies with hyperbilirubinaemia and normal haemoglobin values.

Resuscitation equipment should be checked before starting while the donor blood is gently warmed to 37°C without breaking the seal. The infant is suitably restrained, kept warm (in an incubator if necessary) and kept under continual observation. Each exchange cycle of 20, 10 or 5 ml according to the state of the infant should be accurately measured and recorded.

Rate should not exceed 1·8 ml/kg/minute so that exchange of twice (180 ml/kg) the baby's blood volume will take at least 100 minutes. Fretfulness may be relieved by the slow injection of 1 ml of calcium gluconate 10 per cent or by slowing or halting the procedure for a time.

Watch carefully for vomiting. If there is cyanosis or sudden collapse, stop procedure and concentrate on resuscitation and aspiration of possibly inhaled material.

NEONATAL INFECTIONS

Between 7 to 15 per cent of newly delivered babies develop some signs of sepsis in the first week or so. As most of these infections are minor and some are viral in origin the widespread use of antibotics should be discouraged. Wherever possible swabs for bacteriological culture must be obtained in case the infection spreads. In prolonged rupture of the membranes swabs from liquor, placenta or vagina may give early information on bacteriological sensitivities.

Simple local remedies which are usually effective are hexachlorophene powder (sparingly) or chlorhexidine for mild umbilical or skin sepsis; 0·5 per cent ephedrine in saline for snuffles, oral nystatin 100,000 units before feeds for oral thrush, and exposure to air for perianal dermatitis. Discharging eyes often clear with regular 2-hourly irrigations of tepid sterile saline. Treat persistent discharge after swabbing with chloramphenicol 0·5 per cent eye drops every 1–2 hours and if this fails tetracycline eye ointment. (Gonococcal ophthalmia may be misdiagnosed if a smear is not taken to demonstrate intracellular diplococci. The gonococcus is notoriously difficult to culture.)

More serious infections such as septicaemia, meningitis, pneumonia, osteitis or urinary infection, may give no localising signs initially but should be suspected if there is any departure from the infant's normal behaviour as regards feeding, bowels, sleep or respiration. Unexplained anorexia, loss of weight, fever or hypothermia, persistent jaundice or tachycardia would also suggest full clinical examination supported by blood and urine cell count and culture, throat and umbilical swabs, and by lumbar puncture if appropriate.

Urinary infection may be confirmed by the presence of pus cells in urine. Isolated bacteriuria is an unreliable index. If there is doubt after routine examination of the urine or if the baby is ill, obtain further specimen by bladder puncture.

CMV, rubella or toxoplasma infection may all produce early and persistent jaundice, often with splenomegaly.

Treatment.—Often the gravity of the infant's condition does not allow waiting for the results of bacteriological sensitivity testing. Such "blind" treatment should include antibiotics likely to be effective against Gram-negative bacilli as well as the

staphylococcus. Parenteral administration is often necessary
initially in a sick infant.

Commonly used antibiotics with their limitations. (Dosage, see
pages 189–194.)

Penicillin:	Especially effective against streptococcal infections. Combines well with kanamycin or gentamicin.
Ampicillin:	Broad-spectrum but resistant *E. coli* and other Gram–ve organisms common.
Kanamycin:	Effective against Gram–ve except *Ps. aeruginosa*. Some staphylococci may show resistance. Can only be given I.M. or I.V.
Flucloxacillin:	Only really effective against staphylococci.
Carbenicillin:	A specific penicillin for use against *Ps. aeruginosa* but resistant strains are becoming frequent. It can only be given parenterally and intramuscular injections are painful.
Gentamicin:	A broad-spectrum antibiotic which is often effective against *Ps. aeruginosa*. It can only be administered parenterally.

J.I.

V
INFECTIONS

PYREXIA OF UNCERTAIN ORIGIN

THE history must include inquiry for contact with specific infectious fevers and recent travel abroad; with children in or from tropical areas exotic disease must be seriously considered. It should also be remembered that certain diseases such as measles assume a more malignant and confusing picture in dark-skinned races.

In an ill child without localising signs the following tests are essential: blood culture, urine for microscopy (supra-pubic aspiration in an infant), white cell count and a chest radiograph. A lumbar puncture may also be indicated subject to the proviso on page 90. In a child who has recently returned from abroad typhoid and malaria are two possibilities and they may present with misleading signs such as pneumonia, diarrhoea, constipation, fits, coma or anaemia.

Typhoid may not show such severe constitutional symptoms as in an adult. Irregular pyrexia, cough, disturbed mental state and abdominal distension, followed by diarrhoea, splenomegaly and rose spots should lead to blood and stool culture, and serological tests. Chloramphenicol is the drug of choice in the acute stage, while ampicillin is useful in the treatment of carriers.

Malaria should be considered in any sick child over 3 months of age who may have been exposed to infection and who presents with fever, anaemia, cough or diarrhoea. Convulsions or coma suggest *P. falciparum* infection causing *cerebral malaria* and immediate specific and anticonvulsant treatment is necessary. Occasional presentation in medical shock (*algid malaria*) requires urgent expansion of plasma volume as well as specific therapy. Immediate thick and thin films, blood for haemoglobin and cross-matching should be taken. Treat at once with specific therapy (see page 81) and by blood transfusion if necessary. (Notifiable disease in U.K.)

TABLE OF INCUBATION AND ISOLATION

	Incubation	Isolation of the Infected Person
Chickenpox (Varicella)	7–21 days (14–15 days usually)	Until one week after the appearance of the rash.
*Diphtheria	1–6 days (2–4 days usually)	Until two consecutive negative swabs from nose and throat have been obtained; in no case for less than four weeks.
*Enteric group	3–23 days	Until convalescence is definitely established, and there have been three consecutive negative stools off treatment.
*Infectious hepatitis	15–40 days	7 days minimum.
*Measles (Morbilli)	7–14 days (10–11 days usually to catarrhal stage)	For not less than 5 days from the date of the appearance of the rash.
Mumps (Epidemic Parotitis)	14–28 days (17–18 days usually)	For not less than 2 weeks from onset—provided that one clear week has elapsed since the subsidence of all swelling.
*Poliomyelitis	5–21 days (7–14 days probably usual)	For a minimum period of 3 weeks.
Rubella	14–19 days (17–18 days usually)	Until disappearance of the rash.
*Scarlet fever	2–5 days	For 10 days of penicillin treatment and until 11th–13th day throat swabs proved free.
*Smallpox (Variola)	10–17 days (14 days to appearance of rash usually)	STRICT ISOLATION until every scab has fallen off, and the skin lesions have healed.
*Pertussis	7–14 days to catarrhal stage. A further 7–14 days to paroxysmal stage.	Until the characteristic spasmodic cough and whoop have ceased for at least 2 weeks; or, in cases of persistent whooping, for not less than 4 weeks from the onset of the spasmodic cough.

At risk (quarantine) time; Add 2 days to incubation period.
* Notifiable disease in U.K.

WORM, PROTOZOAL AND CANDIDAL INFECTIONS

Parasitic infections in Great Britain are becoming more common owing to immigration and the extent and rapidity of modern travel. No history is complete without asking if the patient has been abroad at any time and if so where. The following list of parasites are either endemic in Britain (†) or are so widespread abroad that they are likely to be seen in immigrants or travellers. There are many other of more local occurrence and it is recommended that any diagnostic problem in a patient with the appropriate history should be discussed with a clinical pathologist. Those helminthic infestations which at some stage are particularly associated with an eosinophilia are marked with an asterisk (*).

Parasite	Diagnosis	Treatment (details see Chapter XI)	Special Features
(a) HELMINTHS Nematodes (*round worms*) Enterobius vermicularis† (*thread worm*)	Ova on peri-anal skin. (Sellotape slides)	Piperazine + senna (Pripsen) Vipyrnium or thiabendazole	Very common and often symptomless.
Ascaris lumbricoides† .. (*common round worm*)	Ova in stools.	Piperazine (Antepar) Piperazine + senna (Pripsen) Mebendazole.	Resembles earthworm. Loeffler's syndrome.
Trichuris trichiura†* .. (*whipworm*)	Ova in stools.	Thiabendazole. Mebendazole.	Inhabits colon. May cause bloody diarrhoea or rectal prolapse.
Ankylostoma duodenale* Necator americanus (*hookworm*)	Ova in stools.	Bephenium (Alcopar). Mebendazole.	Common in immigrants; often causes serious blood loss (iron & protein).
Toxocara spp.†* .. (*dog and cat round worms*)	Skin and serological tests. Histology: eye, liver & lung.	Diethylcarbamazine (see literature). Thiabendazole.	Visceral larva migrans; history of close contact with puppies; pica.
Trichinella spiralis†* ..	Skin and serological tests. Muscle biopsy (e.g. deltoid).	Piperazine & thiabendazole. Steroids.	History of eating raw pork sausages; fever, myalgia, orbital oedema.
Strongyloides stercoralis* ..	Larvae excreted intermittently.	Thiabendazole. Pyruvinium pamoate.	Pneumonic signs; diarrhoea, abdominal pain.
Cestodes (*tape worms*) Taenia saginata† .. (*beef tape worm*)	Segments in stools.	Niclosamide (Yomesan). Mebendazole.	No risk of cysticercosis.

WORM, PROTOZOAL AND CANDIDAL INFECTIONS—(Continued)

Parasite	Diagnosis	Treatment (details see Chapter XI)	Special Features
Hymenolepis nana	Ova in stools.	Niclosamide (Yomesan). Mebendazole.	Common in Asians—probably symptomless.
Echinococcus granulosus (hydatid) ..	Clinical. Serology and C.F.T. Scolices and hooklets in surgical material (hydatid "sand").	Surgical; symptomatic.	History of contact with dogs in sheep-farming areas.
Trematodes (flukes) Fasciola hepatica .. .. (sheep liver fluke)	Watercress eating. Tender hepatomegaly. Ova in stools.	Emetine hydrochloride.	Can occur in U.K.
(b) PROTOZOA Entamoeba histolytica† ..	C.F.T. Vegetative amoeba in dysenteric stool immediately after passing. Cysts in formed stool in carrier or case of amoebic abscess.	1. Acute amoebiasis—parenteral emetine hydrochloride. 2. Subsequent eradication of intestinal infection—oral treatment with various drugs (EBI, arsenicals, diodoquin, antibiotics). 3. Liver abscess—Chloroquine.	Most cases in patients recently resident in the tropics, but fatal amoebiasis has occurred in those who have never left Britain. At least 6 consecutive negative stool specimens must be obtained before a patient can be considered cured.
Giardia lamblia†	Cysts and flagellates in fresh loose stool and duodenal specimens. Cysts in formed stool.	Metronidazole (Flagyl)	Chronic diarrhoea and malabsorption.
Toxoplasma	Positive Dye Tests and C.F.T. occur in 20-40% of "normal adults" at titres of 1/8-1/128 and in 1% at 1/256. Even a low titre signifies past infection. Fetal titre may exceed maternal in passive immunisation. IgG of maternal origin has a three week half-life. Therefore repeat maternal and fetal titres at six weeks.	Pyrimethamine and Sulphadimidine. Spiramycin (see literature). Steroids.	Neonatal hepatitis, micro- or hydrocephalus, retinitis, uveitis or microphthalmia. Ocular toxoplasmosis: usually congenital and sole lesion. Seen relatively late with visual problem when primary lesion inactive and positive dye test titres in normal range. Acquired toxoplasmosis: meningoencephalitis or pseudo-glandular fever.

WORM, PROTOZOAL AND CANDIDAL INFECTIONS—(Continued)

Parasite	Diagnosis	Treatment (details see Chapter XI)	Special Features
MALARIA Plasmodium falciparum (malignant tertian malaria)	Thick and thin blood films.	Chloroquine (intravenous, and also dexamethasone in cerebral malaria). Quinine. Amodiaquine.	May present as P.U.O. with jaundice, diarrhoea or as encephalitis; rapid killer. Opinion of experienced pathologist needed as soon as possible.
P. vivax, P. ovale, P. malariae (benign tertian and quartan malaria)	Thick and thin blood films.	Clinical cure: Chloroquine, amodiaquine. Radical cure: Chloroquine + primaquine.	Benign relapsing course. Radical cure with primaquine necessitates treatment in bed with certain precautions. Risk of crisis in G-6PD deficient subjects.

Multiple-drug-resistant *P. falciparum* (S. America, S. E. Asia) is best treated with quinine followed by pyrimethamine and sulfadoxine. Suppression for all types of malaria: give either pyrimethamine weekly or proguanil hydrochloride daily. Continue suppression for at least four weeks after leaving endemic area.

CANDIDOSIS

Topical infection	Presence of hyphae in smear. Culture.	Nystatin, amphotericin or clotrimazole preferred to gentian violet (½ %).	After antibiotic therapy. Immune defect.
Systemic infection	Culture of blood and removed prosthesis, etc.	Amphotericin.* Clotrimazole. 5-fluorocytosine (5-F.C.).	Complicates renal dialysis, ventriculocardiostomy, cardiac prostheses, etc.

*Toxicity (esp. renal) and difficulties in administration of amphotericin suggest that oral experimental drugs being tried may be preferable. Clotrimazole (Bayer Pharm. Ltd) at up to 100 mg/kg/day commonly causes gastro-intestinal or mental disturbances but treatment can often be continued. 5-F.C. (Roche) may cause marrow or liver depression but with normal renal function and on 200 mg/kg/day, toxicity appears low.

VIRUS INFECTIONS

RUBELLA

All girls should receive rubella vaccine even though serology would show that 80 per cent are immune in the U.K. Do not give during pregnancy.

Embryopathy risk in maternal rubella is 50 per cent in the first month falling to a low level in the fourth month. Precise history of specific contact and presence of H.A.I. antibody within the incubation period proves past infection. Interpretation depends on precise history and serial titres. Gamma globulin even in high dosage offers very little protection and therefore therapeutic abortion should be considered.

Fetal Rubella

High H.A.I. antibody titres and virus excretion persist for months or years but by 5 years a high antibody titre ($> 1/64$) is consistent with past postnatal infection. A mother immune before pregnancy transfers her antibody across the placenta, leaving the normal neonate with a titre often higher than her own but lower than in fetal infection and falling to zero in early infancy. The presence of cord blood IgM suggests, but its absence does not exclude, fetal infection.

VACCINIA

As deaths from vaccinia exceed those from smallpox in the U.K. vaccination is no longer a D.H.S.S. recommendation, but the primary procedure is safest in the 2nd year. Maternal vaccination may cause fetal death at any gestational period. Vaccination should be avoided during steroid or cytotoxic therapy. Patients with eczema may develop eczema vaccinatum and patients with hypogammaglobulinaemia, vaccina gangrenosa. Vaccination of a child with eczema must be accompanied by antivaccinial gamma globulin. The risk to a child from a vaccinated sibling is low if the lesion is covered by an occlusive dressing.

N.B. Herpetic lesions can simulate eczema vaccinatum and must be distinguished by electron microscopy as treatment differs.

VIRUS INFECTIONS AND THE NEWBORN

The immunity status of the newborn and his risk of cross-infection in the family

Contact with infected mother or sibling	Maternal history of disease known to confer fetal immunity	Gamma globulin[1] recommended for		Separate neonate from infected person
		neonate	other susceptible sibs	
Hepatitis				
(a) infectious	—	YES[2]	YES if has other disease	YES
(b) serum	—	NO	NO[3]	NO
Herpes simplex				
(a) primary	YES	YES	NO	YES
(b) secondary	YES	NO	NO	YES
Measles (or vaccination)	YES	YES	YES	YES
Mumps	NO	YES	if he has other disease[4]	NO
Poliomyelitis	YES	YES	YES	YES
Rubella	NO[5]	NO[6]	NO	NO
Vaccinia (see text)				
Varicella/H. zoster	NO	NO	NO[7]	YES
Variola	NO	YES[8]	YES[8]	YES

1. Seek expert advice regarding dosage.
2. H.G.G. ineffective if given within two weeks of potential clinical onset (see p. 78). As infectious hepatitis is common usually subclinical in children, use of expensive H.G.G. in prophylaxis is reserved for those who have some other disease simultaneously.
3. Cross-infection risk in serum hepatitis is small except for staff handling blood samples, etc.
4. Cachexia, severe congenital heart disease, primary tuberculosis, cystic fibrosis of pancreas, hypogammaglobulinaemia, post-splenectomy steroid or cytotoxic therapy. H.G.G. 250 mg 2–3 days after active immunisation or within 7–10 days of contact modifies the infection but permits an active immunity.
5. Serological evidence only acceptable.
6. Specific anti-rubella H.G.G. available.
7. Malignancy, steroid and cytotoxic therapy may lead to fatal viraemia. Withdrawal of drugs early in the incubation period preferable to increased steroid dosage. Post-zoster H.G.G. may be available.
8. Post-vaccination H.G.G. if available.

The Table has been adapted from *Neonatal Emergencies and Other Problems* (1972) by kind permission of Dr. John Black and the publishers, Butterworth & Co.

Antivaccinial gamma globulin is useful in eye (lid) infections (1 per cent drops half-hourly), eczema vaccinatum and smallpox but not for post-vaccinial encephalitis. Dosage is 0·5–2 g according to age in prevention, but is repeated for treatment.

Methisazone is also of use in the treatment of eczema vaccinatum.

HERPES

For keratitis idoxuridine 0·1 per cent drops once hourly by day and twice hourly at night. The treatment of encephalitis with this agent is disappointing. Extensive superficial lesions can be treated with idoxuridine in dimethylsulphoxide.

SUGGESTED IMMUNISATION SCHEDULE

(Avoid intramuscular injections in children with bleeding disorders).

Age	Vaccine
Newborn	BCG (Recent family history of tuberculosis or immigrant children at risk. Assess nodule at 6/52)
6 months	Diphtheria, tetanus, whooping cough, poliomyelitis: 1st dose*
8 months	Diphtheria, tetanus, whooping cough, poliomyelitis: 2nd dose
12 months	Diphtheria, tetanus, whooping cough, poliomyelitis: 3rd dose
13 months	Measles
15 months	(Smallpox)
School entry	Diphtheria, tetanus, poliomyelitis: 4th dose
10–13 years	BCG if tuberculin negative
11–14 years	Rubella (all girls)
School leaving	Tetanus, poliomyelitis: 5th dose.

*By starting this programme at 6 months, the adverse effect of maternal antibodies and infant maturity on the immune response are avoided.

Pertussis Immunisation

The true incidence of cerebral reactions is uncertain. Immunisation should be deferred during febrile illness and never given to infants with an existing CNS disorder, a history of epilepsy or possible cerebral reaction to a previous dose. Previous local reactions are not a contra-indication.

TETANUS PROPHYLAXIS

1. **Active Immunisation**

   Surgical toilet of the wound is of prime importance. In addition adsorbed tetanus toxoid should be given if: the child has received an incomplete course of immunisation or has not received a booster within the last 5 years.

2. **Passive Immunisation**

   Category A. If the wound is clean, non-penetrating, with negligible tissue damage and less than 6 hours old, antitoxin is not usually recommended.

   Category B. If the wound is more serious or treatment is delayed treat initially as under item 1. A dose of human tetanus antitoxin should be given in the opposite limb to that in which tetanus toxoid was given. A dose of tetanus antitoxin should also be given to those children whose immune status is unknown and in those who received an incomplete course or a booster over 10 years ago.

3. Inform the patient's general practitioner, suggesting a complete course of active immunisation in those who have not previously been immunised.

R.H.G.

[NOTES

VI
PAEDIATRIC EMERGENCIES

GENERAL ADVICE

A rapid history and examination of the seriously ill child should precede emergency treatment either in the admission room or in the ward. The parents must be asked to wait.

Once the initial treatment has been started the parents will be available to give a fuller history which may well be of the utmost importance regarding specific therapy in the early stages. Proper recording of temperature (low reading if necessary), pulse respiration and weight must be made.

DEHYDRATION

Depending on the cause, symptoms may be diarrhoea, vomiting, refusal to feed or polyuria leading to apathy, coma, or fits.

Signs are loss of skin turgor, sunken fontanelle or reduced eye-ball tension. Factual evidence of recent loss of weight may be available from a clinic weight card.

Differential Diagnosis

1. *Gastro-enteritis of infancy.*—Fulminating cases may present before diarrhoea occurs. Rectal examination may produce the obvious evidence of a projectile watery stool and auscultation of abdomen may show either the squeaky protests of an irritated bowel or the almost complete silence of impending ileus with its serious implications.

More commonly vomiting and diarrhoea occurs in infants with a gradual onset and less severity. Such babies if under 5 per cent dehydrated (see p. 47) can often be treated at home with oral replacement of fluid loss.

"Clear fluids" and not antibiotics are the essentials of treatment. There is no evidence that oral antibiotics shorten the illness or reduce the incidence of carriers. The simpler the treatment the better, especially if it is to be carried out at home. Either 5 per cent dextrose (1 level teaspoonful of sugar to 4 oz of water) alone or 4 per cent dextrose and 0·18 per cent saline from an intravenous bottle should be given orally. Unless the salt can be rigorously controlled there will be an unacceptable risk of hypertonic dehydration (see p. 51).

The infant should be offered small amounts frequently (even hourly if necessary) to provide a fluid intake of up to

180 ml per kg for the first 24 hours. If vomiting persists or the stools do not abate in frequency and dehydration increases then admission to hospital for intravenous therapy (p. 47) will be needed.

Usually after 24 hours the clinical condition improves and the child will be able to tolerate quarter-strength formula feeds which can be strengthened daily to half, three-quarters and then full strength.

2. *Other acute infections with anorexia and fever.*—E.g. bronchiolitis, otitis media, pyelonephritis or meningitis. Before performing lumbar puncture its contra-indications must be considered. (See page below).

3. The frequency of *other causes* varies with the age of the child. E.g. diabetes mellitus, adrenal insufficiency either congenital or apoplectic, some forms of poisoning (see page 113) and in hot weather cystic fibrosis with heat stroke.

Treatment—see page 47.

CONVULSIONS AND COMA

These two major symptoms often occur together and may share a similar aetiology. The initial treatment differs only in that fits must be brought rapidly under control to minimise anoxic brain damage.

Emergency treatment consists of clearing and maintaining the airway with the patient lying on his side. Oxygen should be administered as necessary. Certain conditions requiring urgent specific therapy such as hypoglycaemia, hypocalcaemia, hypomagnesaemia, pyridoxine deficiency or alkalosis must be excluded if necessary by therapeutic trial. Seizures must then be controlled by parenteral anticonvulsant therapy such as phenobarbitone, diazepam or paraldehyde. If seizures are not rapidly controlled with moderate doses of parenteral drugs, or if cyanosis persists, the patient should be intubated and ventilated to prevent hypoxia. After prolonged hypoxia cerebral oedema should be anticipated and treated (see page 121).

Differential Diagnosis

1. *Usually with accompanying fever and meningism.*—The causes include meningitis, encephalitis or other infections of varying severity, including *P. falciparum* malaria and Sonne dysentery. **A lumbar puncture may be needed to differentiate**

them but if the history is longer than three days or there is the slightest evidence of chronically raised intracranial pressure a neurosurgeon should be consulted *beforehand*. The CSF pressure should always be measured and if raised, with a clear fluid, the neurosurgeon must be informed immediately so that steps to prevent the likely "cone" can be initiated forthwith.

2. *Usually without meningism or fever.*—Examples are status epilepticus, head injury (battered baby—see page 153), cerebrovascular accident or tumour and these should only be subjected to lumbar puncture after consultation with an experienced doctor.

3. *Cerebral abscess.*—As these cases have longstanding raised intracranial pressure they must not be subjected to the risk of lumbar puncture but as they sometimes present with signs of meningitis the temptation is very real. If the history is longer than a few days or there are signs of chronic sepsis (ear or chest) a neurosurgical consultation is advisable so that diagnosis and treatment of this responsive condition may be safely conducted.

4. *Other causes* are hypertension (in nephritis), poisons such as lead, drugs like corticosteroids and antidepressives. Phenothiazines may cause oculogyric crises.

RESPIRATORY EMERGENCIES*

Ensure a clear airway and give oxygen.

1. Upper airway Obstruction

Presents with stridor due to such causes as epiglottitis, laryngeotracheobronchitis, foreign body, congenital laryngeal stridor.

Epiglottitis should be distinguished from the other causes by its rapid onset over a few hours, associated with a high temperature and a severely ill child. It is associated with a septicaemia due to group B haemophilus influenzae. The patient has difficulty in swallowing and oral feeds are contraindicated. Inspection of the throat may precipitate a respiratory arrest and should only be performed with an anaesthetist at hand. Do not sedate. Take blood cultures, and treat with antibiotics and intravenous fluids. Intubation is indicated in all patients unless constantly observed by an anaesthetist.

*See Roberts, K. D., and Edwards, J. M. *Paediatric Intensive Care*, p. 162 (2nd edit. 1975). Oxford: Blackwell Scientific.

If facilities for the nursing of patients with naso-tracheal tubes are inadequate, tracheostomy is indicated. Both nasal and tracheostomy tubes must be adequately humidified.

2. Lower Airway Obstruction

Presents with wheeze and expiratory rhonchi. Causes include asthma, bronchiolitis (see below) and foreign body.

3. Other Causes of Respiratory Difficulty

(a) *Pulmonary* causes include lobar emphysema, pneumothorax, mediastinal emphysema, staphylococcal pneumonia.

Pneumonia and cystic fibrosis should be treated with oxygen, antibiotics and sedation, and may be helped by inhalations of acetylcysteine before physiotherapy. Artificial ventilation is often unhelpful and is contra-indicated in staphylococcal pneumonia and cystic fibrosis.

(b) *Cardiac.*—Heart failure can easily be missed and is sometimes precipitated and masked by an infection. The heart rate and the size of the liver are important guides (see page 106).

(c) *Metabolic acidosis.*—Deep, sighing respirations should raise the possibility of diabetes mellitus (smell of acetone), aspirin poisoning, "uraemia", periodic syndrome or fulminating infections such as meningococcal septicaemia or gastro-enteritis.

ACUTE BRONCHIOLITIS

This condition is often preceded by an upper respiratory infection followed by failure to feed, increasing dyspnoea and paroxysmal cough. Clinical signs in the chest may be minimal but generalised inspiratory crepitations, emphysema and expiratory wheeze are often found. The chest X-ray shows emphysema only, unless secondary atelectasis or pneumonia has occurred.

Treatment

Oxygen.

Maintain airway free from excess secretions by frequent suction.

Maintain hydration by tube feeding if necessary, parenteral fluid is necessary if vomiting occurs or if gastric distension hinders respiration.

Broad-spectrum antibiotics if secondary bacterial invasion is suspected.

Undue restlessness may require sedation (chloral hydrate or amylobarbitone) but CO_2 retention or hypoxia must first be excluded.

Treatment for heart failure may be required in severe cases, see page 106.

If adequate aspiration of secretions is impossible, if the consciousness level deteriorates, or if the PCO_2 progressively rises or is over 8kPa (60 mmHg), endotracheal intubation should be considered. A general anaesthetic is normally required. Bronchial lavage followed if necessary by "continuous positive airway pressure" or artificial ventilation results in recovery in most cases, but should be performed by experienced personnel.

STATUS ASTHMATICUS

Status asthmaticus in infants and young children produces an increase in the work of respiration, arterial hypoxaemia and metabolic and respiratory acidosis. Baseline values of acid-base balance and PO_2 should be obtained if available.

Immediate Treatment*

DO NOT use the same bronchodilator which the child may have received by any route within the preceding 4 hours. Give oxygen if cyanosed. Avoid sedation or aminophylline suppositories.

Give:
Nebulised salbutamol (if available)
0·5 ml of 0·5 per cent solution diluted with 5 ml saline via Wright's nebuliser with gas flow of 8 litres/min or:
Aminophylline I.V. 4 mg/kg over 10 minutes or:
Salbutamol I.V. 5 µg/kg over 10 minutes or:
Adrenaline S.C. 0·01 ml/kg of 1: 1000 solution.

Follow-up Treatment

If child has not substantially improved on above treatment

*With acknowledgement to Dr. S. Godfrey.

set up I.V. drip of 4·3 per cent dextrose in 0·18 per cent saline if not already started and continue at rate of 70–120 ml/kg/day.

Give:
Hydrocortisone I.V. 2 mg/kg stat followed by 1·0 mg/kg/hr reducing to 0·5 mg/kg/hr when response occurs, and
Aminophylline I.V. 0·7 mg/kg/hr, together with nebulised salbutamol as above 6-hourly.

X-ray chest to exclude pneumothorax or pneumonia; antibiotics need not be given unless infection is likely.

Later treatment

As soon as the child can take by mouth start:
Oral prednisone 0·5 mg/kg 6-hourly, oral salbutamol 0·15 mg/kg 6-hourly or nebulised salbutamol as above 6-hourly.

Steroid therapy to be tapered over five days when clinical improvement has occurred. Previous outpatient treatment should be reviewed and modified before discharge.

Treatment of respiratory failure.

This is indicated by:

1. Severe inspiratory retraction with reduced ventilation which may mask the audible signs of bronchospasm.

2. Deterioration in the level of consciousness.

3. Respiratory acidosis with Pco_2 in excess of 8 kPa (60 mmHg).

4. Hypoxia with arterial Po_2 less than 9·3 kPa (70 mmHg) in 40 per cent oxygen.

If these signs persist after adequate hydration, oxygenation and drug therapy, mechanically assisted ventilation in an intensive therapy unit should be considered.

ACUTE COLLAPSE IN INFANCY

Important Causes

Most commonly this is due to overwhelming infections such as gastro-enteritis or Gram-negative septicaemia, rarely congenital adrenal hyperplasia. A petechial rash would make the diagnosis of meningococcal septicaemia likely.

Clinical features are those of rapid onset of profound shock, extreme pallor, cold extremities, mottled cyanosis, unobtainable blood pressure and acidotic respirations.

Immediate Resuscitation

Ensure a clear airway.

Commence intravenous therapy with either plasma, blood or dextran. If none of those is immediately available use 0·9 per cent saline. Rate: 20 ml/kg by intravenous shot.

If no improvement give hydrocortisone 100 mg/kg intravenously. In the presence of severe disseminated intravascular coagulation (DIC) heparin may also be considered (see p. 177).

Essential Investigations—having achieved an adequate circulation:

Full blood count and platelets—if platelets low, screen for DIC. Blood urea and electrolyte concentrations. Before antibiotic treatment is started investigations such as blood culture, lumbar puncture (warning, see page 90), rectal swab and throat swab must be carried out. Obtain urine specimen with the aid of a plastic bag but do not delay treatment for this.

Further treatment will depend upon the findings *BUT:*

Ensure that a complete fluid balance chart is kept.
Anticipate the development of cerebral oedema (see p. 121).

ADRENOCORTICAL CRISIS

Adrenocortical failure may occur in children who are, or have been, on long-term corticosteroid therapy (including topical steroids) and in babies suffering from the salt-losing variety of congenital adrenal hyperplasia (CAH).

Long-term Therapy

Children should be withdrawn gradually from treatment and it is reasonable to provide ACTH stimulation during the withdrawal period (40 i.u. twice weekly).

The pituitary-adrenal axis may remain depressed for as long as 2 years after steroid therapy over which period any operation or severe illness requires replacement therapy. (See page 197).

Salt-losing Syndrome

Babies suffering from CAH present with an adrenocortical crisis in the second or third week of life. The abnormal external genitalia and the determination of nuclear chromatin should provide an easy diagnosis in girls. The prompt diagnosis in boys is difficult (pigmented nipples and scrotum, low Na, high K). Biochemical diagnosis in both sexes requires the determination of serum androgens and plasma 17-hydroxyprogesterone or if these are not available the determination of the 11-oxygenation index in the urine, the measurement of pregnanetriol and 17-oxosteroid excretion.

Treatment

Whatever the cause of the crisis treatment is urgent. It requires, at first, the rapid intravenous infusion of 0·9 per cent saline with glucose, together with hydrocortisone. Hydrocortisone 100 mg should be given intravenously at once and may be repeated at 2–6 hourly intervals depending on progress at all ages. Inadequate therapy is a common fault, both as regards sodium and hyrocortisone. Even babies may require 3 to 5 g of sodium chloride daily and a salt-retaining hormone should be given. Oral 9 alpha-fludrohydrocortisone 0·1 mg for a baby is appropriate, more for an older child. Hypoglycaemia (page 68) may remain unrecognised and untreated. Infusion therapy should be maintained for 1–2 days. Oedema and hypertension are the signs of excessive therapy.

Maintenance therapy should be trebled prophylactically if sufficient infection or stress occurs.

ACUTE RENAL FAILURE

Acute renal failure usually presents with severe oliguria but is occasionally diagnosed in the presence of a normal urine output, especially when caused by severe burns. It may occur as a complication of four main conditions:

1. Hypovolaemia or hypotension, as in blood loss, dehydration, septicaemia, burns and the nephrotic syndrome.
2. Renal tubular poisoning.
3. Glomerular disease as in glomerular nephritis or the haemolytic-uraemic syndrome.
4. Bilateral renal vein thrombosis, mainly in dehydrated patients.

Most causes are potentially reversible and all types should be treated energetically with recovery in view.

Three phases are recognisable: (i) Potentially reversible oliguria (pre-renal failure). (ii) Established renal failure. (iii) Diuresis.

Treatment depends on the stage in which the patient is first seen. In all cases where acute renal failure is suspected palpation of the abdomen for an enlarged bladder should suggest urinary obstruction (commonly posterior urethral valves in boys).

Catheterisation is generally necessary initially, for diagnostic purposes, but an in-dwelling catheter should be avoided because of the risk of infection. A plain abdominal X-ray should be taken to assess renal size and exclude calculi.

The following data should be obtained immediately: Body weight, serum electrolytes, osmolality, urea, creatinine, calcium acid base status, haemoglobin, haematocrit and blood for group and cross-match.

1. Potentially Reversible Oliguria

Vigorous treatment to remove underlying cause, i.e. hypovolaemia, dehydration or obstruction. Dehydration should be assessed (see p. 47) and corrected as rapidly as possible with an isotonic fluid. If the random urine: plasma (U : P) urea ratio is 5 or more and the U : P osmolality ratio 1·1 or more, the oliguria is physiological and will respond to rehydration. If oliguria ($<$ 200 ml/24 hours/m^2) persists after rehydration and the U : P urea and osmolality ratios are low, the patient should be given mannitol 0·75 g/kg (e.g. 3·5 ml/kg of a 20 per cent solution) intravenously in 5 minutes followed if necessary by frusemide 5 mg/kg intravenously 15 minutes later. If there is still no diuresis, confirmed if necessary by bladder catheterisation, management for established renal failure must be started *immediately* to prevent fluid overload.

Pre-renal oliguria due to the nephrotic syndrome requires completely different management. Here, the hypovolaemia is compensated by sodium retention but may be severe enough to cause significant azotaemia with serum albumin levels $<$ 10 g/l. *Large doses of frusemide should be avoided* because the salt and water diuresis induced may precipitate acute renal failure. It is more logical to correct the plasma protein deficit by infusing albumin, bearing in mind the very real hazard of cardiac failure from a too sudden plasma volume expansion. The following regime is satisfactory when carefully supervised:

Salt-poor albumin, 0·5 g/kg by intravenous infusion over approximately 1 hour; followed by frusemide, 2 mg/kg intravenously.

The effect is transient owing to continuing proteinuria, but the schedule may be repeated at 6-hourly intervals, as required.

2. Established Renal Failure

Successful management demands careful attention to the following:

(a) *Fluid requirements*

The daily fluid requirement is the sum of:
(i) Extrarenal insensible loss less water derived from metabolic processes. Allow 15 ml/kg in infants, 12 ml/kg in older children. This value should be increased by 10 per cent for each 1°C fever present.
(ii) Gastro-intestinal losses.
(iii) Urine output. In practice the preceding day's urine output is used. Fluid balance should be recorded as accurately as possible but frequent weighing is the only reliable guide. With proper management, tissue break-down will cause a daily weight loss of the order of 0·5 per cent of body weight.

(b) *Electrolyte requirements*

Sodium: No significant urinary loss will occur during oliguria. Gastro-intestinal losses, i.e. diarrhoea and vomiting, must be replaced by a fluid of similar electrolyte composition, see page 50.

Potassium: A steady rise in the serum level occurs from protein catabolism and cellular disruption. No additional potassium should be given during the oliguric phase. The ECG provides a valuable guide to impending toxicity. For emergency treatment of cardiotoxic effects, correct acidosis and give (i) I.V. glucose 4 g/kg with 1 unit soluble insulin/4 g glucose; (ii) calcium gluconate 10 per cent, 0·3 ml/kg; (iii) resonium A 0·5 g/kg orally or rectally. These will control the hyperkalaemia for 3–4 hours until dialysis can be arranged.

(c) *Calorie and protein requirement:*

Both are necessary to reduce catabolism and delay azotaemia and hyperkalaemia. 50–100 cals/kg/day should be given mainly as concentrated carbohydrate (Hycal and Caloreen by mouth) and fat (intravenous preparations or oral Prosparol). The limiting factors are volume and palatability. At least 0·5 g/kg/ day of high-class protein, e.g. egg or low-sodium milks, should also be given.

(d) Drugs

Prophylactic antibiotics are not indicated. Many drugs are excreted largely by the kidney and dosage should be controlled by measurement of blood levels. When this is not possible, normal doses should be given at increased intervals which are determined by the metabolism and routes of excretion of each drug.

Indications for Dialysis

If oliguria is prolonged or the child is intensely hyper-catabolic, as in massive burns or septicaemia, clinical and metabolic deterioration may occur despite careful conservative management, and dialysis is required. The indications vary in individual patients and the following is only an approximate guide.

Serum potassium greater than 7 mmol/l, or ECG changes.
Blood urea greater than 40 mmol/l (240 mg/100 ml)
Plasma bicarbonate less than 13 mmol/l.
Uncontrolled hypertension.
Overhydration—oedema and weight gain.
Progressive clinical deterioration e.g. drowsiness, convulsions.

Peritoneal dialysis is generally used but, in certain instances, e.g. peritonitis, abdominal wall burns, haemodialysis is indicated. The former is comparatively simple and cheap, but is undoubtedly safer and more effective in the hands of larger paediatric units with special facilities for treatment and monitoring.

HYPERTENSIVE CRISES

Severe hypertension may be caused by sodium overload or by renin/angiotensin excess in both acute and chronic renal failure. For encephalopathy or when the diastolic B.P. is over 120 mm Hg, intravenous diazoxide 5 mg/kg should be used and repeated as necessary. Subcutaneous pentolinium, intra-muscular reserpine or intravenous hydrallazine are also effective. If oral therapy is possible bethanidine or methyldopa should be given and repeated six-hourly. Their effect is potentiated by thiazide diuretics, e.g. bendrofluazide 5–10 mg daily. Dialysis to remove sodium and water is indicated in oliguric patients with hypertensive encephalopathy or heart failure.

DIABETES MELLITUS

DIABETIC KETOACIDOSIS AND DEHYDRATION

Coma or pre-coma may be the presenting feature of diabetes or may occur in a known diabetic due to poor insulin control or to infection. The child should be admitted as QUICKLY AS POSSIBLE and the laboratory warned to expect blood samples.

Initial Management

Weight: assess dehydration (5–10–15 per cent; see p. 47) and send blood for urgent glucose (fluoride tube), electrolytes and Astrup determinations; look for infection; aspirate stomach.

Intravenous Fluids

Of major importance in treatment.—Initially infuse half of the calculated loss from dehydration plus one-quarter of the day's basal requirements, given as 0·9 per cent saline, over the first six hours of treatment. Reassess fluid input two-hourly in relation to dehydration, urine output and vomit.

If blood hydrogen ion (H^+) concentration equals more than 80 mmol/l (pH less than 7·1) or standard bicarbonate concentration less than 12 mmol/l give one-third of calculated sodium bicarbonate according to the formula for non-respiratory acidosis (page 49). This should be divided between bottles; if large volumes of sodium bicarbonate are given the normal saline solution may need to be reduced in concentration to half or three-quarter normal strength.

Potassium

This should be given from the start of treatment if there is not proven oliguria. Initially 6 mmol/kg/day and not more than 20 mmol/l of infusate. Ideally potassium should be given with ECG monitoring of the "T" waves.

Insulin (1) Standard, or (2) Continuous

(1) *Standard regime*: On admission in ketoacidosis give soluble insulin 0·5 units/kg (half I.V. and half I.M.).

In all cases it is essential to repeat the blood sugar estimations about two hours after the first dose of insulin and when the result is available give further soluble insulin as follows:

Blood sugar the same: repeat initial dose at once*

Blood sugar falling: wait until 4 hours after the initial dose then give half this intramuscularly.

Blood sugar rising: give twice the initial dose immediately*.

The half-life of insulin intravenously is 5 minutes, intramuscularly is 2 hours, and subcutaneously it is variable. Because of this an alternative regime using continuous intravenous insulin may be used. However, a constant infusion pump is necessary to ensure that an unvarying amount of insulin is given to the patient.

(2) *Alternative insulin regime for ketoacidosis:* If this method is to be used an initial bolus dose of soluble insulin 0·05 unit/kg is given followed by 0·05 unit/kg/hour until the blood sugar is less than 14 mmol/l (250 mg/100 ml). The rate of insulin infusion may be rapidly altered depending upon the fall in blood sugar concentration. To make up the insulin solution: withdraw 5 ml of blood from the patient into a 50 ml syringe; add insulin requirements for 8 hours and make up to 50 ml with sterile normal saline (blood is required to prevent insulin binding to the syringe).

Subsequent Management after Initial Control by Either Regime

When blood sugar concentration less than 14 mmol/l (220 mg/100 ml) change to 4 per cent dextrose in 0·18 per cent saline and oral potassium supplement.

Oral feeding can usually begin about 12 hours after admission with small (15–30 ml) quantities hourly. Fluids should include glucose (about 20 g 3-hourly).

Most children can then be controlled by giving soluble insulin 4-hourly, adjusting the dose according to the result of urine testing. Example—24 kg child:

If the peripheral circulation is still poor give half the dose intravenously.

Urine Sugar				Soluble Insulin Dose
	2 per cent with acetone	..	..	12 units
	1 per cent with acetone	..	..	10 units
or	2 per cent without acetone	..	..	
	1 per cent	..	..	..	8 units
	¾ per cent	..	..	..	6 units
	½ per cent	..	..	..	4 units
	Nil	..	..	..	2 units

The sliding scale may later be given 6-hourly then 8-hourly.

Note: *Hypoglycaemia* is possible whilst the patient is still ketotic and drowsy. Watch for signs such as sudden change of level of consciousness, irritability, sweating, convulsions, extensor plantar responses. If it is *suspected* take blood for sugar estimation and give 30–60 ml of 50 per cent dextrose *immediately* by vein.

WITHOUT SEVERE ACIDOSIS OR DEHYDRATION

Most children are in this group at the time of diagnosis and stabilisation can usually be achieved by the following regime:

Insulin

A rough guide to the size of the initial dose is 0·5 units per kg subcutaneously. Thereafter insulin is given three times daily before breakfast, lunch and supper according to urine tests (see above). Some insulin will be necessary when urine tests are negative. Parental education in the administration of insulin should begin at this stage.

When the urine is free from ketone bodies and moderate stabilisation is achieved a mixture of equal quantities of crystalline and amorphous insulin zinc suspension is given once daily before breakfast. The combined dose approximates to 3/4 of the total amount of soluble insulin given the previous day. The doses of the two insulins are then adjusted as necessary to achieve optimal hospital control.

Diet

The daily calories are apportioned approximately as follows:

Carbohydrate 40–45 per cent, protein 15–20 per cent, fat 35–40 per cent. The carbohydrate intake is regulated through the day, the basis for the calculation being the quantity of each item of food which contains 10 g of carbohydrate (= 1 portion). The total daily portions of carbohydrate are divided into roughly equal amounts for breakfast, lunch and supper with "snacks" of roughly 10–20 g (1–2 portions) for mid-morning and 30–40 g (3–4 portions) at tea time.

About 1000 calories per day are necessary at one year, increasing by approximately 100 calories per day for each year of age until puberty. The calorie content of the diet should be decided before discharge but final stabilisation of insulin dosage is only possible at home.

Hypoglycaemic Action of Insulins
(subcutaneous administration)

	Onset of Action	Peak Action	Dura- tion
Crystalline (soluble)	1 (hour)	2–4 (hours)	6–8 (hours)
Semi-lente (Amorphous I.Z.S.)	$1\frac{1}{2}$–2	5–7	12–18
Isophane (N.P.H.) Insulin	1–2	10–20	20–32
Lente (I.Z.S.)	$1\frac{1}{2}$–2	14–18	26–30
Ultra-lente (Crystalline I.Z.S.)	5–8	22–26	34–36
Actrapid (Monocomponent)	$1\frac{1}{2}$–1	3–5	7
Semitard (Monocomponent)	$1\frac{1}{2}$	5–9	15
Monotard (Monocomponent)	3	7–14	22

Monocomponent pork insulins are less antigenic and the dose required is usually $\frac{2}{3}$–$\frac{3}{4}$ of other insulins.

Standard insulin syringe: 1 mark = 1 unit of 20 units/ml insulin.

CONGENITAL HEART LESIONS AND CARDIAC EMERGENCIES

Newborn babies going into heart failure or showing progressive cyanosis need urgent investigation. Once symptoms develop deterioration is often rapid and a few hours' delay may prove fatal. Immediate referral to a paediatric cardiology centre is advised as open heart surgery, when necessary, is now possible at any age or weight.

Acyanotic conditions liable to cause signs of heart failure and respiratory distress in infancy commonly include coarctation of the aorta and left-to-right shunts.

Cyanotic congenital heart conditions commonly include transposition of the great arteries, Fallot's tetralogy and tricuspid atresia.

Arrhythmias.—Paroxysmal tachycardia is the commonest arrhythmia in infants. The heart rate is rapid and regular. Although digoxin is usually effective it should not be used as it might render later DC countershock hazardous. Initial treatment may include the cautious, slow intravenous injection of propranolol, verapamil or mexiletine (see literature for dosage) under careful ECG and blood pressure monitoring. The "cardiac arrest" team should be standing by.

Ventricular arrhythmias are uncommon and can be recognised only by electrocardiography. They are treated by intravenous lignocaine or procainamide. In resistant cases phenytoin, quinidine or a beta-blocking agent should be tried.

Congenital heart block may occur without other cardiac abnormality but more commonly is associated with a defect such as corrected transposition, Ebstein's anomaly or myocarditis. The condition rarely requires treatment but a persistently slow pulse rate (usually less than 40 per minute) may cause heart failure or syncopal attacks and should then be treated by intravenous isoprenaline (2–4 mg in 500 ml of 50 g/l dextrose) infused fast enough to increase the rate to about 80 per minute. Alternatively cardiac pacing by intravenous electrode can be used.

The table (*opposite*) gives the dose in micrograms 2 × *daily* for maintenance and the relevant volumes of the elixir and the injection to deliver that amount.

In the rare instances where digitalisation is needed more urgently, 2½ × the maintenance dose may be given orally or by injection and half this amount might be repeated once, 8–12 hours later, before continuing with the maintenance dose.

Please note that there are three different strengths of liquid preparation. Elixir digoxin *paediatric*, 50 mcg per ml, Inj. digoxin *paediatric*, 100 mcg per ml and Inj. digoxin B.P. 250 mcg per ml.

DIGOXIN DOSAGE

Patients weight in kg	Maintenance oral/I.M. dose at 5 mcg/kg twice daily			Maximum single intramuscular or intravenous dose i.e. Two-and-a-half times maintenance dose for digitalisation		
	mcg per dose	Elixir Digoxin 50 mcg in 1 ml No. of ml	Paed. Inj. Digoxin 100 mcg in 1 ml No. of ml	mcg per dose	Paed. Inj. Digoxin 100 mcg in 1 ml No. of ml	Inj. Digoxin B.P. 250 mcg in 1 ml No. of ml
1·0	5·0	0·1	0·05	12·5	0·125	0·05
1·5	7·5	0·15	0·075	18·75	0·187	0·075
2·0	10·0	0·20	0·10	25·00	0·25	0·1
2·5	12·5	0·25	0·125	31·25	0·312	0·125
3·0	15·0	0·30	0·15	37·50	0·375	0·15
3·5	17·5	0·35	0·175	43·75	0·437	0·175
4·0	20·0	0·40	0·20	50·00	0·50	0·2
5·0	25·0	0·50	0·25	62·5	0·625	0·25
6·0	30·0	0·6	0·30	75·0	0·75	0·3
7·0	35·0	0·7	0·35	87·5	0·875	0·35
8·0	40·0	0·8	0·40	100·0	1·0	0·4
9·0	45·0	0·9	0·45	112·5	1·125	0·45
10·0 (1 year)	50·0	1·0	0·50	125·0	1·25	0·5
15·0 (3 years)	75·0	1·5	0·75	187·5	1·875	0·75
20·0 (5 years)	100·0	2·0	1·0	250·0	—	1·0
25·0 (8 years)	125·0	2·5	0·5 (adult strength)	250·0	—	1·0
50·0 + (Adult)	250·0	250 mcg (adult tablet)	1·0 (adult strength)	500·0 mcg = 0·5 mg	—	2·0

P.V.M.—9

HEART FAILURE

The usual symptoms in infancy are respiratory distress with panting after feeds, anorexia and failure to thrive. Enlargement of the liver, rapid breathing, tachycardia, and oedema shown by weight gain or puffiness around the eyes, are the usual signs. In such cases, the heart is usually enlarged on X-ray.

Treatment

All infants in heart failure should be considered for referral of a paediatric cardiology centre for possible operative correction of an underlying congenital heart lesion.

Initially the following manoeuvres may be tried.
1. Semi-upright nursing.
2. Oxygen.
3. Tube-feeding.
4. Diuretics—frusemide is the most effective.
5. Digoxin.
6. Potassium supplement.

Oxygen should be administered while these measures are being taken.

CYANOTIC ATTACKS

These attacks are particularly common in children with Fallot's tetralogy. They are characterised by shortness of breath, increasing cyanosis, tachycardia and perhaps loss of consciousness or a convulsion. As the condition deteriorates the systolic murmur becomes fainter and shorter and may disappear. The child should be nursed in the knee/elbow position. Intravenous propranolol should be given at a rate not exceeding 0·25 mg every minute. (See page 182.) The drug should be stopped if there is a significant fall in blood pressure or pulse rate. Oxygen should be administered while these measures are being taken. It is important to avoid dehydration in all types of cyanotic heart disease because of the danger of vascular thrombosis.

Antibiotics

Antibiotic cover must be given to all children with congenital and rheumatic heart disease if teeth are to be extracted or an operation is undertaken; 300,000 units of procaine penicillin should be given at the time and should be followed by oral penicillin, 250 mg four times daily for one week. If the child is on prophylactic penicillin and a tooth has to be extracted a different antibiotic (e.g. erythromycin) should be given.

Children with rheumatic heart disease need continuous penicillin prophylaxis to reduce the likelihood of relapse (penicillin V, 125 mg twice daily).

CARDIAC ARREST

The commonest cause of a "cardiac arrest call" is a respiratory arrest with a secondary cardiac arrest. Causes include inhalation of vomit, anoxia, anaesthetics and other drugs, hyperkalaemia, and as a result of serious arrhythmias during cardiac catheterisation.

Immediate Action

Summon emergency team, clear airway and maintain ventilation by mouth-to-mouth respiration or endotracheal intubation until anaesthetist arrives. Start external cardiac massage: place child on firm surface, compress sternum with heel of hand, rhythmically 50–60 times per minute. Success judged by feeling temporal pulse. Aspirate pharynx intermittently and continue until emergency team arrives.

Emergency Team

Anaesthetist is usually responsible for ventilation, while another doctor should continue cardiac massage. Nurse prepares cutdown trolley. Give sodium bicarbonate I.V. Assume base deficit of 20 mmol in infants, 30–40 mmol in older children. After Astrup determination, if metabolic acidosis persists give further bicarbonate according to formula on page 49.

Cardioversion.—Connect machine to mains and leads to patient. Record ECG on oscilloscope. If asystole is confirmed (straight line of oscilloscope) try to induce ventricular fibrillation by giving 2–3 ml of 1 : 10,000 solution of adrenaline and calcium gluconate 2–3 ml of 100 g/l solution or calcium chloride 100–200 mg intravenously or into the heart before preparing for manual external shock. Use 50–70 Joules initially for small infants and 100–250 Joules for older children, depending on size and age. Drugs should not be given into the heart if the patient is on positive pressure ventilation as this may precipitate a pneumothorax. Failure to restore sinus rhythm after defibrillation may be due to anoxia (check ventilation), metabolic acidosis (corrected by more bicarbonate) or a very irritable myocardium (tall, coarse ventricular fibrillatory waves on the oscilloscope) or insufficient Joules (use higher energy). In resistant cases of coarse ventricular fibrillation use lignocaine 10 mg or propranolol 1 mg or phenytoin sodium 5–10 mg intravenously or into the heart before attempting further DC shock with higher energy. If fine ventricular fibrillation persists with low voltage fibrillatory waves on ECG give adrenaline or calcium chloride before attempting further defibrillation. In some cases of asystole or resistant ventricular fibrillation transvenous pacing may be needed.

Resuscitation should be continued for as long as the patient responds or ECG evidence of cardiac depolarisation persists. (Dilated unresponsive pupils or flat EEG are ominous signs.)

Ventricular arrhythmias are common after resuscitation and are usually due to metabolic acidosis, anoxaemia or digoxin.

Treatment consists of correcting the acidosis and using a suitable anti-arrhythmic agent such as lignocaine, procainamide, phenytoin or a beta-blocking agent.

P.R.B.

EXTENSIVE BURNS

Anoxia is the first complication to consider, especially if the face has been burned or the child has been in smoke. Causes are laryngeal obstruction, pulmonary oedema, contracted burned skin encircling the chest, carboxyhaemoglobin, anaemia and shock. If oxygen and humidification are not adequate, positive pressure ventilation will be needed.

If possible weigh the patient before treatment is started. Sedation is not indicated unless the child complains of continuing pain: papaveretum (see page 179) or heroin (0·1 mg/kg) can be given intravenously. Prescribe tetanus toxoid (0·5 ml I.M.) to the actively immunised; a 7-day course of systemic erythromycin estolate or cloxacillin to the unprotected; and human anti-tetanus globulin (A.T.G., "Humotet" Wellcome) (1 ml I.M.) if treatment has been delayed, or the wound is heavily contaminated with soil or faeces. A urethral catheter should be passed if the burn is over 25 per cent.

If the burn extends over more than 10 per cent of the body surface, excluding erythema (i.e. one whole upper limb), the child will need intravenous therapy to prevent or correct shock. Colloid (plasma, plasma protein fraction, or dextran 110 in saline) is better than electrolyte solution alone but they can be given in equal proportions. Plasma equal to the child's plasma volume (see page 133) should be given for every 15 per cent of skin burned, one-half in the first 8 hours, and the other half in the next 16 hours. This rate should be adjusted to keep the capillary haematocrit near normal and the urine output at 1 ml/kg/hour. Water by mouth should be limited to three-quarters of the normal intake (see page 18). Blood is rarely needed in the shock stage but can be given at the end of it (usually an amount equal to 20–40 per cent of the blood volume for burns over 40 per cent). During the shock stage one should look for evidence or renal failure, which may be oliguric or non-oliguric.

If parts of the burn are deep, a surgeon should see the case early with a view to excision and skin grafting on the third or fourth days. (Analgesia to pin-prick signifies a deep dermal burn or full thickness skin destruction). Early excision for a child under 3 years of age is not generally advised: blood loss is always great and up two blood volumes may be needed.

At the end of the shock stage (48 hours) food should be started. If oral feeding is not accepted, potassium should be given without further delay by mouth or intravenously in a generous amount to prevent ileus (see page 47).

The burn is a fistula leaking water, sodium and potassium. The rate of water loss through it averages 0.30 ml/cm² burned area/day. The average sodium loss is 0.03 mmol/cm² burned area/day. The protein loss is similar to dilute plasma, about 30 g/l. Extensively burned patients probably need $1\frac{1}{2}$ times the calories and 2–3 times the protein needed in health and this should be achieved over several days.

D.C.J.

VII

ACCIDENTAL POISONING

Poison Information Centres in U.K.

Telephone Numbers:
London 01-407 7600   *Leeds* 0532-32799
Cardiff 0222-33101   *Belfast* 0232-30503
Newcastle-upon-Tyne 0632-25131 *Edinburgh* 031-229 2477

The usual age group is 1–4 years with the maximum incidence around 2. Boys outnumber girls 2:1. Drugs, of which aspirin is the commonest, account for the majority of cases, the remainder are mainly household substances.

INITIAL MANAGEMENT

Measures which are relevant to the treatment of all poisoned patients are the maintenance of an adequate airway, the removal and identification of the ingested substance and the management of any complications (supportive treatment). Whatever treatment is given should be carried out calmly and methodically, the indiscriminate use of antidotes, sedatives or stimulants can be more dangerous than the poison. Time should not be wasted giving universal antidote. Specific antidotes are mentioned in the appropriate sections.

Removal of the Ingested Poison

Stomach emptying is best achieved by vomiting; however emesis should not be induced in the unconscious patient or after ingestion of corrosives (phenols, alkalis) or paraffin (kerosene).

Methods

Immediate—push a finger or spoon handle down the throat, easier if preceded by a drink of water or milk.

Ipecacuanha Paediatric Emetic Draught 10–15 ml followed by 1–2 glasses of water. The dose can be repeated after 15 minutes but if vomiting does not occur within 10 minutes lavage must be performed. It is ineffective after the ingestion of antiemetics, phenothiazines, atropine and amphetamines.

Gastric lavage should never be attempted on the unconscious patient without prior insertion of a cuffed endotracheal tube.

113

It is not recommended after ingestion of paraffin (aspiration, lipoid pneumonia), or corrosives (perforation).

Method: wrap the child in a restraining sheet and lay on the left side. Tilt the table head down. Choose a tube with a large lumen (at least 28 F.G., 17 E.G.) and mark the distance from the bridge of the nose to the xiphisternum. Lubricate with water-soluble jelly. Pass by mouth to the mark. Make sure the tube is not in the trachea (coughing, continuous bubbling) and always aspirate for stomach contents before starting lavage. Lavage with 150–200 ml amounts of warm isotonic saline, 1 per cent sodium bicarbonate or tap water (note risk of water intoxication) and continue until the returned fluid is clear.

Purges and enemata may remove unabsorbed material from the gut but can add to the irritant effect of the poison. A solution of sodium sulphate 300 mg/kg is recommended.

Osmotic diuresis with mannitol 10 per cent 2 g/kg I.V. or hypertonic solutions of urea or dextrose will increase excretion of various poisons but may cause dangerous hypokalaemia if potassium-containing fluids are not administered. The excretion of salicylates and barbiturates is enhanced when osmotic diuresis is combined with an alkaline urine. Amphetamine excretion is enhanced in an acid urine.

Exchange transfusions have been used in poisoning by salicylates, iron, chlorinated hydrocarbons, copper sulphate.

Peritoneal dialysis and haemodialysis are of value if the poison is diffusible and the toxicity is related to the blood concentration, e.g. barbiturates, salicylates. Indications are deep coma, apnoeic episodes, hypotension and oliguria.

Identification

The container and label should be obtained if possible. Tablets can be checked for colour, size and code against charts. The prescriber, dispensing chemist, manufacturer or Poison Information Centre can provide information. These procedures are far quicker than analysis of specimens. When uncertain save (in order of usefulness) specimens of:

Vomitus or first gastric aspirate.
Urine—particularly if some hours after ingestion.
Venous blood.

Supportive Treatment

Recordings of temperature, pulse, respiration, blood pressure and fluid intake/output should be routine.

Temperature regulation.—Hyperpyrexia (over 40°C) should be treated by exposure, cold-water sponging and fans.

Hypothermia—cover with warmed blankets. The use of heat lamps, hot water bottles and pads can be dangerous if the patient is unconscious.

Pain should be adequately treated with analgesics.

Delirium and excitation. Chlorpromazine I.M. is recommended.

Antibiotics should be used to treat specific infections only.

Other measures are dealt with in the following sections: circulatory failure (page 94), respiratory failure (page 91), fluid and electrolyte balance (page 47), acidosis (page 49), convulsions and coma (page 90), nutrition (page 21), hypoglycaemia (page 68) and acute renal failure (page 96).

SPECIFIC POISONS

Salicylates

Peak blood levels are reached between 2 and 3 hours after ingestion. Fifty per cent of ingested aspirin is excreted in the first 24 hours. 150–200 mg/kg of aspirin will cause symptoms.

Symptoms.—Initial hyperventilation produces respiratory alkalosis and renal compensation increases the urinary loss of base. This phase is usually short in children and is followed by metabolic acidosis. Carbohydrate metabolism is disturbed causing ketosis, rarely hypoglycaemia. Dehydration, hyperpyrexia and hypoprothrombinaemia may also occur.

Investigations.—Serum salicylate—a level below 2·92 mmol/l (40 mg/100 ml) rarely causes symptoms, over 8·76 mmol/l (120 mg/100 ml) is usually lethal.

Blood H^+ concentration, Pco_2, standard bicarbonate, electrolytes, blood sugar and prothrombin time.

Urine gives a mauve to violet colour with Phenistix and violet with $FeCl_3$ persisting after boiling.

Treatment.—Gastric lavage with 1 per cent sodium bicarbonate or emesis, even if more than 4 hours after ingestion.

Press oral fluids. Dextrose saline should be given I.V. if the child is vomiting or collapsed (100–150 ml/kg/24 hours).

Bicarbonate corrects the metabolic acidosis (page 49). It should not be given intravenously without estimating blood H^+ concentration. Alkalinising the urine increases the excretion of salicylate (2 mmol bicarbonate/kg should normally raise urine pH to 7 or more). In severe ketoacidosis bicarbonate may cause hypernatraemia; additional potassium should be given, provided renal function is adequate.

Acetazolamide 5 mg/kg given orally or I.M. 6–8-hourly also increases urinary salicylate excretion.

Hypoprothrombinaemia may be corrected by vitamin K_1 I.M. or I.V. and by transfusions.

Avoid giving CNS depressants, e.g. barbiturates, morphine.

Alkaline osmotic diuresis, dialysis or exchange transfusion may be required.

Paracetamol

Hepatic damage, often not evident for several days after ingestion, is a life-threatening complication of overdosage. Vomiting, gastro-intestinal haemorrhage, hyper- or hypoglycaemia, renal tubular damage and cerebral oedema may occur. Management is supportive following stomach emptying and induction of a diuresis. Peritoneal dialysis is ineffective, but haemodialysis may be necessary if renal failure develops.

Iron

The principal effects are gastro-intestinal fluid loss with corrosion and haemorrhage, shock and liver damage. The vomit appears rusty and has a characteristic metallic smell. The presence of ferrous salts in the vomit can easily be confirmed by the Prussian Blue (ferricyanide) test. The serum iron is raised but does not correlate well with the severity of intoxication.

Treatment is urgent. Immediate gastric lavage with 1 per cent sodium bicarbonate, some being left in the stomach (see general management).

Desferrioxamine should be given in the presence of gastro-intestinal symptoms, shock, altered consciousness or the ingestion of an obviously toxic quantity of iron (e.g. > 40 mg elemental iron/kg ≏ 200 mg ferrous sulphate/kg).

    (a) 500 mg to 1 g in 5 ml water is given I.M. as soon as possible (before lavage).

(b) 5 g in 50–100 ml water is left in the stomach after lavage.
(c) 15 mg/kg/hour is given I.V. if the patient is collapsed, the maximum dose being 80 mg/kg/24 hours.
(d) Up to 2 g I.M. may be given 12-hourly if necessary.

Supportive treatment, in particular fluid balance, is vital. In severe cases shock may occur 16–24 hours after ingestion. After recovery severe gastro-intestinal scarring may occur.

Psychotropic Drugs (Barbiturates and other Sedatives)

The chief dangers are respiratory depression and shock. Hypothermia, water loss from skin and lungs, reduction in urine volume, hypostatic or aspiration pneumonia and cerebral oedema may occur.

Treatment.—The management of pulmonary ventilation and shock comes first. Gastric lavage is usually required but the child who is merely drowsy should be allowed to sleep off the effects under observation. Alkaline osmotic diuresis (see salicylates), dialysis or exchange transfusion may be necessary. Analeptic drugs should not be used.

Tricyclic Antidepressants (Imipramine)

Ingestion of 10 mg/kg or more causes neurological disturbances, respiratory depression and cardiac dysrhythmias. Gastric emptying should be carried out. Drowsiness occurs, often alternating with periods of excitement, convulsions may be controlled with phenobarbitone or diazepam; if respiratory depression is marked, paraldehyde is preferred. Circulatory collapse may occur up to three days after ingestion. ECG monitoring is essential; atropine-like effects of the drug cause tachycardia, but direct toxic effects on the myocardium may cause ventricular arrhythmias, a-v block, hypotension and QRS changes. Pyridostigmine (up to 0·5 mg) by slow I.V. injection has been shown to reverse cardiotoxic effects, propranolol and lignocaine may suppress arrhythmias; hypertensive drugs are not advisable. Peritoneal and haemodialysis are ineffective, but osmotic diuresis may be tried.

Phenothiazines

Overdosage causes hypotension, hypothermia, tachycardia, cardiac arrhythmias, convulsions, and extrapyramidal reactions. Disturbances of consciousness and respiratory depression are less marked than with other sedatives. The stomach should be emptied using lavage since emetics are of little value in this situation. Treatment is supportive and symptomatic. Severe dyskinesia may be treated with anti-parkinsonian drugs (benztropine mesylate 0·1–0·25 mg I.M.) or antihistamines (diphenhydramine hydrochloride 2·5–5·0 mg I.M. or slowly I.V.).

Atropine Group

The usual sources are travel sickness pills (hyoscine) and berries (the nightshades). Symptoms are flushed, hot, dry skin, dilated pupils, tachycardia, hyperpyrexia, urinary retention, delirium and coma.

Treatment.—Gastric lavage, sedation with chlorpromazine I.M., control of body temperature and high fluid intake. Pilocarpine 0·1 mg/kg I.M. or S.C. will counter the peripheral effects but not the more serious CNS ones.

Amphetamines

Amphetamines cause cerebral stimulation with restlessness, tachycardia, irritability, hallucinations, delirium and convulsions followed by profound depression.

Treatment.—Gastric lavage and sedation with chlorpromazine. Osmotic diuresis with acidification of the urine to pH 5·3 or less using ammonium chloride 75 mg/kg effectively increases excretion.

Alcohol

Severe hypoglycaemia may develop several hours after the ingestion of alcohol by small children.

Treatment.—Gastric lavage. Oral or intravenous glucose prophylactically. If the blood sugar is low give 30–50 ml 50 per cent dextrose I.V. followed by an I.V. infusion of 20 per cent dextrose.

Household Products

Caustic alkalis are used in drain cleaners, paint removers and some water softeners. Ingestion causes intensely painful burns of the mouth, pharynx and oesophagus. The mucosa looks soapy white, later becoming brown, oedematous and ulcerated. Perforation of the oesophagus or respiratory obstruction from laryngeal oedema and inability to swallow secretions may occur. Oesophageal stricture may develop after recovery.

Supportive treatment is more important than specific measures. Emesis or gastric lavage are not advisable and could cause perforation of the oesophagus. Attempts to neutralise or dilute the alkali with milk, water, or orange juice are usually unhelpful as the burn is immediate. Oesophago-scopy within 12 hours of injury is advised. If the oesophagus is burnt, broad-spectrum antibiotics should be given and gastrostomy considered. Corticosteroids may prevent the development of a stricture but their use is controversial. Early transfer to a thoracic surgical unit is recommended.

Bleaches are usually solutions of hypochlorites which are corrosives. Give 30 ml aluminium hydroxide gel or magnesium hydroxide. The affected skin should be washed thoroughly.

Soaps, detergents and oral contraceptives are mild gastric irritants. Specific treatment is not required.

Paraffin (Kerosene) and Petroleum Distillates

Symptoms are due to pulmonary irritation (which can be fatal) and CNS depression.

Removal by vomiting or lavage may cause aspiration and neither procedure is recommended. Liquid paraffin (mineral oil) 50 ml by mouth will delay absorption. Corticosteroids and antibiotics may be of value in lipoid pneumonia.

Paraquat and Diquat

Liquid preparations produce intestinal, renal and hepatic damage and particularly delayed pulmonary fibrosis which is progressive and irreversible. Even small quantities are lethal. The onset of symptoms may be delayed for 2–3 days. Urine for analysis (consult Poison Bureau) should be deep-frozen.

Treatment.—Induce vomiting immediately followed by careful gastric lavage. A 30 per cent suspension of Fuller's earth B.P. given *within* 30 *minutes of ingestion* may delay absorption. Promote excretion by prolonged forced diuresis (see p. 114) (10 ml urine/minute/1·73 sq m body surface area). Supportive therapy for hepatic and renal failure may be re-quired.

Plants

Children frequently eat unidentified berries or toadstools. A common problem is laburnum seeds which may cause nausea, vomiting, diarrhoea and collapse.

Treatment is gastric emptying and supportive.

Chronic Lead Poisoning

The usual sources are paint, toys and contaminated water, occasionally the fumes or ashes of burning batteries. Absorbed lead is deposited mainly in the bones but the brain, liver and other viscera may be involved. It is a cumulative poison and is only slowly removed by treatment.

Symptoms are variable and often insidious. Pallor and pica are common. Vomiting, anorexia, abdominal pain or constipation may occur. Encephalopathy, common in children, may present suddenly with convulsions, coma and signs of raised intracranial pressure or gradually with drowsiness, ataxia, irritability, overactivity and retarded development.

Investigations.—A raised whole blood lead (page 138) is usually diagnostic of lead poisoning.

None of the tests mentioned below is specific.

Blood findings are basophilic stippling of the red cells and an iron deficiency anaemia which is rarely severe.

X-rays show a line of increased density at the metaphyses of the long bones. The gut may contain radio-opaque material.

Urinary coproporphrin and Δ amino-laevulinic acid excretion are increased provided lead has been ingested within a week of testing. Glycosuria and aminoaciduria (tubular damage) may occur.

Faeces. The presence of lead or flecks of paint suggests recent ingestion.

CSF. The pressure and protein may be raised. Cells, mainly lymphocytes, are usually below 100/mm³.

Treatment should be started without delay if the diagnosis is suspected.

Any unabsorbed lead should be removed from the gut by gastric lavage, saline purge and enema if necessary before starting specific treatment.

Sodium calciumedetate (calcium disodium versenate) forms a non-toxic chelate with lead which is excreted in the urine. The dose is 70 mg/kg/24 hours, divided into two doses, diluted with dextrose saline and given intravenously over a period of 1 hour. Each course should not exceed 5 days and should be followed by an interval of at least 2 days before repeating.

Dimercaprol (BAL) may be combined with sodium calciumedetate in acute encephalopathy. The dose is 4 mg/kg I.M. 4-hourly for up to 5 days. Toxic effects such as fever, salivation, burning pains and agitation occur rapidly after injection and may be reduced by ephedrine or antihistamines.

Penicillamine is a less toxic chelating agent and is effective by mouth. It is used after the acute phase or if the child is not seriously ill. The suggested dose is 250 mg daily below 5 years old, 250 mg twice daily from 5–10 and 750 mg to 1 g daily over 10. Treatment should be continued for 6–8 weeks or until blood and urine lead levels are normal.

In acute encephalopathy supportive treatment and an adequate urine output are vital. Convulsions should be treated with intravenous diazepam.

Cerebral Oedema

Raised intracranial pressure is due to cerebral oedema and may be reduced by mannitol 20 per cent 2 g/kg given I.V. over 30–60 minutes. Dexamethasone is also effective, the initial dose is 4 mg I.V. followed by 4–8 mg daily I.M. or I.V. in divided doses for up to 2 weeks with a gradual reduction thereafter.

Before the child is discharged home the source of lead must be removed. It is wise to examine siblings and friends.

M.J.B.

[NOTES]

VIII
DIAGNOSIS AND MANAGEMENT
OF
HAEMATOLOGICAL DISORDERS

Diagnosis.—Leukaemia in childhood is predominantly acute lymphoblastic in type, less then 20 per cent of cases are acute myeloblastic or myelomonocytic. Although blast cells may circulate in the blood the diagnosis should be confirmed by demonstrating bone marrow replacement with leukaemic cells. Cytochemical techniques should be used to confirm the cell type, if this is in doubt, before antimitotics are given.

General.—At diagnosis, or subsequent relapse, the patient is at risk from septicaemia and/or bleeding. Take blood cultures when febrile, especially if neutropenic, and use a broad-spectrum antibiotic combination immediately if there is any suspicion of infection. Intramuscular injections must not be given in the presence of thrombocytopenia. When there is severe thrombocytopenia and bleeding give fresh whole-blood or platelet concentrate (see p. 133). Follow-up bone marrows at 2–3 month intervals will detect early haematological relapse and allow treatment to be changed before the patient again becomes at risk from neutropenia or thrombocytopenia. Plot blood count results and the treatment given on semi-logarithmic haematological charts (available from: Wightman Mountain Ltd., 32–34 Great Peter Street, London, S.W.1. Reference No. BMJ 22870).

Varicella and measles may be fatal. If contact with these infections occurs, give hyperimmune gamma globulin within 72 hours: for varicella, zoster immune globulin 1 g/m^2 I.M., for measles, non-specific gamma globulin in similar dose, depending on potency of batch.

Specialist Treatment of Acute Lymphoblastic Leukaemia

Whenever possible newly diagnosed untreated cases should be referred to a specialist centre for accurate classification of cell type, for intensive therapy and for prophylactic cranial irradiation to prevent the subsequent development of CNS leukaemia.

(a) *Drugs used for remission induction and re-induction*

Prednisolone—40 mg/m^2/day by mouth over 3 weeks, tailing to stop in week 4.

Vincristine—1·5 mg/m² once weekly intravenously for 3–4 injections. Ensure a clean venepuncture and flush with 5 ml of saline before and after the injection, using a scalp-vein needle in the hand, cubital fossa or foot. Give methylcellulose (see page 178) to prevent vincristine-induced constipation.

Asparaginase—10,000 units/m² on alternate days × 4, in the third or fourth week of treatment. Have hydrocortisone at hand in case of anaphylaxis.

Always give allopurinol (see page 171) during remission induction to prevent uric acid nephropathy.

(b) Drugs used for maintenance of remission

Bone marrow examination should be considered in order to confirm remission state (less than 5 per cent marrow blast cells) before maintenance therapy is started.

Intensive treatment with one of the effective multi-drug regimes is given for 2–3 years, and then, if no relapse has occurred, treatment may be stopped. Methotrexate, 6-mercaptopurine, vincristine, prednisolone, cyclophosphamide, etc. are used simultaneously or in sequence in maximum tolerable dosage. Treatment should be stopped temporarily if the neutrophil count falls below 1·0 × 10⁹/l or the platelet count below 100 × 10⁹/l, and during serious infections. Folinic acid (24 mg/m² 8-hourly) is the specific antidote to methotrexate.

Treatment of Acute Myeloblastic/Monocytic Leukaemia

Combination chemotherapy in high dosage with resulting marrow aplasia is usually required to attain remission. The following drug combination may be used in centres with adequate support facilities:

Daunorubicin—55 mg/m²/day intravenously on day 1
plus
Cytosine arabinoside—70 mg/m²/day intravenously
on days 1–5.

Repeated 5-day courses should be given with 5-day intervals between courses until remission is obtained. The same combination, given at monthly intervals, may be used for maintenance.

Meningeal leukaemia.—This serious complication develops in at least 50 per cent of patients with lymphoblastic leukaemia who do not receive any form of prophylactic treatment.

After haematological remission, for prophylaxis give:

2400 rad to the cranium over 3 weeks together with once weekly intrathecal methotrexate (10 mg/m^2 but not exceeding 12 mg) for 4 or 5 injections.

For treatment

If a patient with leukaemia develops recurrent headache or vomiting or shows disproportionate weight gain or papill-oedema a lumbar puncture should be performed and, if leukaemic cells are found, intrathecal methotrexate should be given (see para above) twice weekly, and then once weekly, until the CSF count is less than 5 × 10^6/l (5/cu mm).

HAEMORRHAGIC DISORDERS

Screening Tests.—Recommended screening tests for sus-pected congenital bleeding disorders and prior to visceral biopsy are given on page 132. An appropriate clinical and family history is equally important; in particular, details of the patient's haemostatic response to previous surgical procedures. The ingestion of aspirin and other drugs and vitamin C de-ficiency should be excluded because a prolonged bleeding time due to abnormal platelet function may result.

Disseminated Intravascular Coagulation.—This may com-plicate meningococcaemia and septicaemia, newborn hypoxia, extensive surgical procedures, liver failure and other conditions with acidosis and shock. Screening tests, which can be per-formed on capillary blood, are given on page 132.

HAEMOPHILIA

Diagnosis.—A sex-linked recessive disorder occurring in males with a prolonged partial thromboplastin time and normal prothrombin and bleeding times. Factor VIII level is reduced below 50 per cent (0–1 per cent = severe; 1–5 per cent moderately severe; above 5 per cent = mild haemophilia).

Treatment of acute episodes.—Prompt replacement therapy with cryoprecipitate-AHG, freeze-dried factor VIII concen-trate or fresh frozen plasma, within a few hours is vital. Delay overnight may convert a mild bleed into a major one, will retard recovery and also encourage joint damage and muscle wasting. Bed rest, local pressure and haemostatics are of minor importance in comparison. Whenever possible the area should be immobilised (e.g. with a plastic or plaster back slab). Admission is usually required for knee haemarthroses, large haematomas which may cause nerve palsies or vascular obstruction, injuries to the head or mouth and suspected intra-abdominal bleeding. Patients should be screened for hepatitis-associated antigen/antibody.

NEVER cut down, never give aspirin or intramuscular injections, and never venepuncture the jugular or femoral veins

Operative procedures including dental extraction must always be performed at Haemophilia Centres because of the need for factor concentrates, laboratory monitoring of plasma levels and pre-operative screening for acquired inhibitors.

Replacement therapy:

Cryoprecipitate-AHG: Number of packs required for minor episodes $= \dfrac{\text{wt (kg)}}{6}$

Fresh frozen plasma: 20 ml/kg intravenously as rapidly as circulation permits.

These preparations are unstable and retain their potency only when deep frozen at $-20°C$; therefore do not thaw until immediately before use.

Freeze-dried factor VIII concentrate (stable until dissolved at room temperature). Dose for minor episodes $= 12$ units/kg daily or 12-hourly according to the nature of bleed.

CHRISTMAS DISEASE

Similar to haemophilia in respect of inheritance and clinical features, but due to factor IX deficiency. Cryoprecipitate-AHG is of no value. Use fresh frozen plasma or freeze-dried factor IX concentrate instead.

VON WILLEBRAND'S DISEASE

An autosomal dominant disorder with a prolonged bleeding time, due to defective platelet function, and usually also a mild reduction in factor VIII level. Haemarthroses are uncommon and mucous membrane bleeding and haematuria are seen more often. Give replacement therapy as in haemophilia.

HAEMOGLOBINOPATHIES

Diagnosis.—Immigrant children (see page 130), should be screened before surgery or if anaemic for the presence of an abnormal haemoglobin by the following tests—haemoglobin level and reticulocyte count, blood film for target cells, solubility test for haemoglobin S, haemoglobin electrophoresis and fetal haemoglobin and haemoglobin A_2 levels (see page 130).

Management

(*a*) **Sickle-cell disease.**—Homozygote (Hb S/S) and double heterozygote (Hb S/C disease, Hb S/Thal) patients should avoid hypoxia, chilling and dehydration. Early treatment of infection and folic acid supplementation are valuable prophylactic measures. When a painful thrombotic crisis develops dehydration should be corrected, any precipitating infection treated, analgesics given, and the patient kept warm. More specific measures (e.g. intravenous magnesium sulphate) are not of proven value when tissue infarction has occurred.

When a surgical procedure under general anaesthesia is required the patient should be pre-oxygenated with 100 per cent oxygen for 5 minutes and the anaesthetic mixture thereafter should contain at least 30 per cent oxygen. Hydration must be maintained with warmed intravenous fluids, hypotension and tourniquets must be avoided, and the patient kept warm. Pre-operative transfusion from the patient's usual haemoglobin level to an arbitrary normal range is not recommended; if transfusion is necessary the blood should be less than 5 days old and warmed during the transfusion. Exchange transfusion should be considered for major procedures.

Sickle-cell heterozygotes (Hb A/S) are unlikely to have symptoms except under conditions of severe hypoxia. Haematuria may occur however.

(*b*) **Hb C, D or E disease.**—The homozygous states of these disorders may cause mild haemolytic anaemia with target cells in the blood film. The heterozygote forms are symptom-free and are not anaemic.

(*c*) **Thalassaemia.**—The β-thalassaemia homozygote (thalassaemia major) is usually dependent on regular transfusions. The haemoglobin level should be maintained above 8·0 g/dl (g/100 ml) using leucocyte-free packed cells. DTPA (2 g) may be added to each unit of blood transfused and daily intramuscular desferrioxamine (500 mg) may be given to delay the onset of transfusion haemosiderosis. Oral iron therapy is contra-indicated but folic acid supplements should be given. Avoid splenectomy unless secondary hypersplenism leads to neutropenia, thrombocytopenia or an increase in transfusion requirements. Check for endocrine effects of excess tissue iron deposition, especially in the pancreas and pituitary.

The β-thalassaemia heterozygote is symptom-free but occasionally shows mild refractory anaemia.

HAEMOGLOBINOPATHIES

Haemoglobin	Geographica origin	Hb level g/dl	Hb electrophoresis	Fetal Hb level %	Hb A$_2$ level %
Normal (over 1 year)	Any	> 10·5	Hb A	< 2	< 3
Sickle-cell homozygote	African American Caribbean } Negro	5–10	Hb S present Hb A absent	5–10	< 3
Sickle-cell heterozygote	Ditto	> 10·5	Hb S and Hb A present	< 2	< 3
Hb S/C disease	Ditto	10–14	Hb S and C present. Hb A absent	< 2	< 3
Sickle/ thalassaemia	Ditto	5–14	Hb S present Hb A absent or much diminished	2–30	< 3
Thalassaemia major	Mediterranean countries India Pakistan Middle East Far East Negro	Transfusion dependent	No abnormal haemoglobin	10–90	Up to 7
Thalassaemia minor	Ditto	> 10·5 or mild anaemia	No abnormal haemoglobin	Up to 7	Up to 10

G-6-PD DEFICIENCY

This sex-linked disorder may occur in homozygous or heterozygous form in the female or in hemizygous form in the male. It is found in the Mediterranean countries, India, Pakistan, the Middle and Far East and in Negroes. Haemolysis may be induced by drugs and chemicals with oxidant properties and by certain infections. A list of prohibited drugs should be issued to the parents and the general practitioner, and also attached to the hospital case record.

Diagnosis.—There are several screening tests for the detection of glucose-6-phosphate dehydrogenase (G-6-PD) deficiency; a positive result should then be confirmed by a spectrophotometric assay of the actual G-6-PD level.

Drugs and Other Agents available in the U.K. which may cause Haemolysis in Children with Red Cell Glucose-6-Phosphate Dehydrogenase (G-6-PD) Deficiency:

Analgesics and Antipyretics
    acetylsalicylic acid (aspirin)   phenacetin (acetophenetidin)
    *phenazone (antipyrine)

Antimalarials
    chloroquine   mepacrine   primaquine

Antibiotics
    chloramphenicol   nalidixic acid   niridazole   PAS
    nitrofurans   sulphonamides   sulphones

Diabetic Acidosis
Infections
    Miscellaneous bacterial and viral infections (e.g. pneumonia, hepatitis, mononucleosis).
    When infections in G-6-PD deficient patients have been treated with chemotherapeutic agents it may be difficult to establish whether the infection or the chemotherapeutic agent precipitated haemolysis.

Miscellaneous agents
    dichloralphenazone   dimercaprol   *fava beans
    methylene blue   naphthalene   probenecid   *quinidine
    vitamin C (ascorbic acid)   vitamin K_1 (large doses of water-soluble preparations)

*Reported to cause haemolysis in G-6-PD deficient Caucasians but not in deficient Negroes.

COAGULATION INVESTIGATIONS

Screening tests for suspected bleeding disorders

	Normal range
Platelet count low	$150–400 \times 10^9/l$
Bleeding time prolonged	up to 7 minutes
Prothrombin time prolonged	within 2–3 secs of control
or	
Thrombotest reduced	70–130%
Partial thromboplastin time with kaolin prolonged	within 6–7 secs of control

Screening tests for suspected DIC

	Normal range
Platelet count low	$150–400 \times 10^9/l$
Blood film shows red cell fragmentation	
Fibrinogen level low	1·5–4·0 g/l
Serum FDP increased	0–10 µg/ml
Factor V assay low	50–200%

ROUTINE HAEMATOLOGICAL VALUES
approximate normal range

Age	Hb g/dl (g/100 ml)	PCV	WCC × 10⁹/l	Neutrophils %	MCV fl	MCHC%
Cord blood	13·5–20·0	0·50–0·56	9–30	50–80	110–128	29·5–33·5
day 1	17·0–21·0	0·55–0·65	9–40	50–80	110–128	29·5–33·5
day 4	16·0–20·0	0·50–0·58	6–20	35–60	10–121	31 –34
week 2	14·5–18·0	0·50–0·55	6–15	30–50	100–120	30 –34
6 months	10·0–12·5	0·33–0·38	6–15	30–50	} 80–96	
1–5 years	10·5–13·0	0·36–0·40	6–15	30–50		
5–10 years	11·0–14·0	0·37–0·42	5–15	40–65		
10–15 years	11·5–14·5	0·38–0·42	4–13	50–75		32 –36

Serum B₁₂ 150–1000 ng/l 〕 5 ml in plain tube
Serum folate 3·0–20 ng/ml 〕
Red cell folate 100–640 ng/ml 2 ml in heparin or sequestrene tube.

Transfusion of Blood Products.
The infant's blood volume is 8 per cent (80 ml/kg) of the body weight, so that a whole blood transfusion of 20 ml/kg will raise the haemoglobin by approximately 25 per cent.
Amount of packed cells required (ml) = Wt (kg) × 3 × desired rise in Hb (g/dl).
The maximum rates recommended for the treatment of coagulation disorders or for transfusing anaemic patients (e.g. thalassaemics and leukaemics) but not for those being transfused after acute haemorrhage, are:
(a) Fresh frozen plasma 20 ml per kg in 30 minutes
(b) Whole blood 〕 2·5 ml per kg per hour
(c) Packed cells 〕 Maximum in one transfusion 50 ml per kg
Platelet concentrate: 1 unit = platelet concentrate from one pint of blood.
1 unit/m² raises platelet count by 10 × 10⁹/l.
To arrest haemorrhage due to thrombocytopenia give at least 4 units/m².

J.R.M.

[NOTES]

IX

CLINICAL CHEMISTRY

AVERAGE BIOCHEMICAL STANDARDS FOR HEALTHY CHILDREN

Specimen. The material preferred for analysis is indicated in brackets: B = whole blood; P = plasma; S = serum.

*Denotes those investigations often collected by laboratory staff or where special preparation or precautions are needed before collecting the specimen. Concentrations of sodium and potassium in some specimens of capillary blood may be increased to a variable extent.

Enzyme activity depends on the method and units used: consult the local laboratory for normal values.

Blood	S.I. Units	Conventional Units (and Conversion factor)	Comments
Acid base (Astrup, B)* pH (Hydrogen ion)	7·36–7·42 (38–44 nmol/l)	—	Values for arterial blood; results from capillary blood from *warmed* limb are similar.
Pco₂	4·3–6·1 kPa	32–46 mmHg (0·133)	
Standard bicarbonate	21–25 mmol/l	—	
Base excess	−2 — 2 mmol/l	—	Newborn period, down to −4 mmol/l.
Po₂	10·6–13·3 kPa	80–100 mmHg (0·133)	Capillary blood: for arterial blood add 0·7 kPa (5 mmHg) to both limits.
Ammonium nitrogen (Fenton method, P)*	2–25 μmol/l	3–35 μg/dl (0·714)	Newborn period, twice as high.
Bilirubin, Total (P, S.)	2–14 μmol/l	0·1–0·8 mg/dl (17·1)	Newborn period, lower.
Calcium (P, S)	2·25–2·75 mmol/l	9–11 mg/dl (0·25)	Avoid venous stasis: correct for serum protein.
Cholesterol (P, S)	2·6–5·7 mmol/l	100–200 mg/dl (0·0259)	Lower in first year.
Creatinine (P, S)	25–115 μmol/l	0·3–1·3 mg/dl (88·4)	Increases with age within this range.
Electrolytes (P, S)			
Sodium	136–145 mmol/l	—	
Potassium	4·0–5·5 mmol/l	—	
Chloride	98–105 mmol/l	—	
Glucose (specific, fasting) (P, B)	2·5–5·3 mmol/l	45–95 mg/dl (0·0555)	Lower in newborn period. Significant depletion shown by 0·2 g/l or less. May be zero up to age 6 m.
Haptoglobin	0·4–2·0 g/l	—	

AVERAGE BIOCHEMICAL STANDARDS FOR HEALTHY CHILDREN—(Continued)

Specimen. The material preferred for analysis is indicated in brackets: B = whole blood; P = plasma; S = serum.

*Denotes those investigations often collected by laboratory staff or where special preparation or precautions are needed before collecting the specimen. Concentrations of sodium and potassium in some specimens of capillary blood may be increased to a variable extent.

Enzyme activity depends on the method and units used: consult the local laboratory for normal values.

Blood	S.I. Units		Conventional Units (and Conversion factor)		Comments
Iron (S)	9–36	μmol/l	50–200	μg/dl (0·179)	High in newborn period, increases with age.
Iron-binding capacity (S)	45–70	μmol/l	250–400	μg/dl (0·179)	
Lead (B)*	less than 1·75	μmol/l	less than 36	μg/dl (0·0484)	
Lipid (Total)	4–8	g/l	—		
Magnesium (P, S)	0·6–1·0	mmol/l	1·5–2·5	mg/dl (0·411)	
Osmolality (P, S)	275–295	mosmol/kg			
Phenylalanine (P)	0·04–0·21	mmol/l	0·7–3·5	mg/dl (0·0605)	
Phosphate, inorganic (as P) (P, S)	1·1–1·9	mmol/l	3·5–6·0	mg/dl (0·323)	Higher in newborn period. Upper limit 25% lower in older children.
Protein (S)					
Total	63–81	g/l	—		
Albumin	36–48	g/l	—		
Globulin	23–37	g/l	—		
Immunoglobulins					
IgA	0·8–4·5	g/l	—		
IgG	5–18	g/l	—		
IgM	0·2–2·0	g/l	—		
IgE	less than 100–500	μg/l			
Protein-bound Iodine (S)	310–590	nmol/l	4·0–7·5	μg/dl (78·8)	
Triglyceride (S)*	0·34–1·92	mmol/l	30–170	mg/dl (0·0113)	
Urate (P, S)*	0·12–0·36	mmol/l	2–6	mg/dl (0·0595)	
Urea (fasting) (P, S)	2·5–6·6	mmol/l	15–40	mg/dl (0·166)	
Urea nitrogen (fasting) (P, S)	—		7–19	mg/dl	
Faeces					
Fat (as stearic acid)	less than 16·2	mmol/d	less than 4·5	g/d (3·52)	
Cerebrospinal fluid					
Protein (Total)	0·2–0·4	g/l	—		
Sugar	2·5–4·8	mmol/l	45–85	mg/dl	

CLINICAL CHEMISTRY

General

Blood specimens, clotted (to yield serum), fluoride-oxalate (for glucose) and heparinised (whole blood or plasma) are usually suitable. For bilirubin, the specimen must be kept in the dark. Many analyses (electrolytes and enzymes) require prompt separation of cells from plasma.

Urine specimens may require appropriate preservatives. 24-hour collections should be complete and even trivial losses reported. The duration of shorter collections should be governed by the times the patient passes urine (noted exactly) rather than by the clock.

Acid-Base Balance (Astrup)

Only arterial balance is useful. Provided there is good peripheral flow, achieved by warming the limb if necessary, capillary blood is suitable. Blood from an arterial catheter may be taken in a heparinised syringe without entrainment of air and the syringe closed by a cap or bending the needle back. The specimen must then be delivered without delay to the laboratory. When abnormal, the patient's rectal temperature should be reported to enable an approximate correction of the results to be made. Results are reported as pH (or hydrogen ion concentration [H^+]), Pco_2, standard bicarbonate and base excess. The Pco_2 measures the respiratory component of acid-base balance. Standard bicarbonate, which is the concentration of bicarbonate in fully oxygenated whole blood when the Pco_2 is 5·3 kPa (40 mmHg) and the temperature 38°C, measures the non-respiratory component. Base excess (which may be negative) is derived from the standard bicarbonate. This may be used to assess the base required for whole body correction, which is equal to the base excess in mmol/l × body wt in kg × 0·3 (The total required is greater than this but the amount derived from this formula will avoid transient dangerously high blood levels.)

Glucose Tolerance

For at least three days before the test the diet must contain adequate carbohydrate. After a 12-hour fast (4 hours for an infant) take capillary blood for sugar determination, then give glucose by mouth, 1 g/kg but never less than 10 g or more than 50 g. At suitable intervals after the glucose has been ingested take further capillary blood specimens for sugar determinations at 30-min intervals for 3 hours. Tests for glycosuria should be made during the investigation.

Hypoglycaemia

The most useful investigation is to collect blood within a few minutes of a clinical manifestation thought to be due to hypoglycaemia. Specific methods for blood glucose should be used.

The following tests may be useful between attacks and involve venous blood collections for glucose (whole blood, fluoride-oxalate tube) and insulin (plain tube, no haemolysis, separate serum with minimal delay and store at $-20°C$).

1. *Determination of fasting glucose and insulin.*—Fast the patient overnight and take blood at 08·00 h for glucose and insulin on three consecutive days, taking blood at the same time on each occasion. Assay insulin only in specimens with a low glucose concentration. Inappropriate insulin secretion at the time of hypoglycaemia is the best index of insulinoma. If basal insulin concentration is normal, proceed to test 2. Test several urine specimens for ketones. This may indicate the occurrence of ketotic hypoglycaemia.

2. *Leucine sensitivity test.*—Facilities for intravenous administration of glucose and hydrocortisone should be available throughout the test. A fasting venous blood specimen is taken for glucose and insulin determination (two or three may be needed in a very unstable patient) and then 0·15 g/kg L-leucine given by mouth. Further specimens are taken for glucose and insulin at 15, 30, 45, 60, 90 and 120 min after the dose.

3. *Glucagon test.*—This test may be used to investigate both glycogen storage disease and insulinoma. For investigating insulinoma this is safer than the tolbutamide test.

Fast the patient for 12 h (in small children for as long as possible) and take capillary blood 20 min and again immediately before giving glucagon intravenously. (Dose, see page 176). Shock following intravenous injection has been reported in a few patients and appropriate precautions should be taken.

For glycogen storage disease further specimens are taken at 20, 40, 60, 90 and 120 min after injection. In addition take venous blood (1 ml) for lactate determination immediately before and 60 min after glucagon. Normally a rise of 2·2 mmol/l (40 mg/100 ml) of glucose or more is obtained. If the response is smaller the test should be repeated 2·5 h after a carbohydrate meal following a day of normal feeds.

For insulinoma all samples should be venous for glucose and, when less than 2·2 mmol/l, for insulin assay. Take blood immediately before and at 5, 10, 15, 30, 60, 90 and 120 min after the intravenous glucagon (same dose, see page 176). Insulin concentrations greater than 100 mU/l are suggestive of an insulinoma.

4. Patients with growth hormone deficiency or hypoadrenalism may present with hypoglycaemia. See below for insulin stimulation and ACTH tests.

Pituitary, Adrenal and Gonadal Function

Nomenclature and abbreviations are confused: the following are recommended:

Trophic hormones: ACTH—adrenocorticotrophin; GH—growth hormone; FSH—follicle stimulating hormone; LH—luteinising hormone (sometimes ICSH—interstitial cell-stimulating hormone; FSH and LH are both gonadotrophins); TSH—thyrotrophin; prolactin.

Releasing hormones: CRF—corticotrophin releasing factor; LH–RH or LH–FSH–RH—luteinising and follicle stimulating hormone releasing hormone; TRH—thyrotrophin releasing hormone.

Inhibiting factors: PIF—prolactin inhibiting factor; SRIF—somatostatin.

The following tests are useful to assess extreme short stature, adrenocortical insufficiency and male hypogonadism.

If growth hormone deficiency is likely, and especially if there is evidence of other trophic hormone deficiencies, the screening test for growth hormone should precede the insulin test and adequate pituitary-adrenal function must first have been demonstrated by showing a normal diurnal rhythm of serum cortisol.

Screening test for growth hormone deficiency.—The patient should fast from 18·00 h the previous evening or for a minimum of 12 h prior to the test. Blood is collected for blood glucose (1 ml in fluoride-oxalate tube) and for growth hormone estimation (plain tube, 2 ml to give 0·5 ml serum).

Glucose, 1·75 g/kg, but not more than 50 g, is then given orally, and further blood samples for glucose and growth hormone collected at 3, 4 and 5 h after the dose. At least one value for serum growth hormone should exceed 10 mU/l for an adequate response.

Insulin sensitivity test.—This test should be used to confirm growth hormone deficiency if suspected from the results of the screening test. A doctor should be in attendance throughout. The patient should fast from 18·00 h the previous evening or for a minimum of 12 h. A polythene cannula is inserted into an antecubital vein and a slow intravenous infusion of normal saline commenced. A three-way tap inserted between the cannula and infusion set allows blood samples to be taken without stress and dextrose or glucagon to be given if severe signs of hypoglycaemia occur. Soluble (crystalline, glucagon-free) insulin 0·1 unit/kg is given intravenously (0·05 unit/kg for children weighing less than 15 kg or with good evidence of panhypopituitarism). Blood is taken for blood glucose, and serum cortisol (3 ml blood to give 1 ml serum) in the fasting state and at 20, 30, 60, 90 and 120 min. In addition glucose is measured at 70 and 30 min.

A fall in blood glucose by 40 per cent of the fasting value at 20–30 min is required for adequate stimulation of the pituitary-adrenal axis. The blood glucose response (insulin sensitivity and hypoglycaemia unresponsiveness) considered alone is an unreliable indication of pituitary function (growth hormone and ACTH release) in childhood. Peak responses of growth hormone and cortisol occur at 60 min after insulin. A value exceeding 10 mU/l for growth hormone should be demonstrable at least once during the course of the test for an adequate response. The peak response of cortisol normally occurs at 60 min after insulin and should exceed 386 nmol/l (14 µg/100 ml).

Diurnal rhythm of serum cortisol.—This is a sensitive index of pituitary ACTH release and adrenal cortisol production. Serum cortisol values are highest between 06·00 h and 09·00 h and lowest between midnight and 04·00 hours. The normal range is approximately 140–552 nmol/l (5–20 µg/100 ml) and samples taken at 08·00–09·00 and 16·00 h should differ by at least 140 nmol/l (5 µg/100 ml).

Short-term ACTH test.—A basal blood is taken for serum cortisol at 10·00 h (1 ml serum). Depot synthetic peptide, tetracosactrin (Synacthen) 0·5 mg is then given I.M. Further samples of blood are taken at 1, 4 and 5 h after the injection for serum cortisol measurement. Normal (basal) ranges for serum cortisol at 10·00 h are 140–552 nmol/l (5–20 µg/100 ml) and peak responses after Synacthen (normally at 4 h) 580–1518 nmol/l (21–55 µg/100 ml).

Long-term ACTH test.—Children suspected of having primary adrenal insufficiency should be tested with Synacthen *depot* over a three-day period and the urinary free cortisol measured.

Day 1: Collect a base-line 24 h urine from 10·00 h without preservative.

On days 2, 3 and 4 give Synacthen *depot* 0·5 mg intramuscularly at 10·00 h and 18·00 h. Collect three 24 h urine samples for analysis of urinary free cortisol. Expected normal values (corrected for body weight) are 5·6 ± 2·8 nmol/kg (2 ± 1 µg/kg) rising to 347 ± 280 nmol/kg (124 ± 100 µg/kg) by the third day.

Human chorionic gonadotrophin (HCG) stimulation test.— This should only be performed on male patients with retarded pubertal development.

Day 1: Collect a basal blood at 10·00 h (3 ml of serum). Give 1500 i.u. HCG (Pregnyl) intramuscularly after basal blood collection.

On days 2, 3 and 4 repeat the injection of HCG (1500 i.u.) and collect further blood on days 3, 4 and 5 for radioimmunoassay of serum androgens. This represents mainly testosterone and closely related biologically active metabolites which cross-react in the assay. Prepubertally, basal levels are normally < 4 nmol/l in boys, rising steadily as puberty intervenes to 15–46 nmol/l in the adult. Responses after HCG are age and maturation dependent; a two-fold or greater increase over basal levels suggests intact Leydig cell function.

Thyroid Function

Normal values are tentative and should be confirmed locally.
Serum thyroxine (T_4) is the preferred *first* measurement in both hypo- and hyperthyroidism. Drugs may decrease T_4,

hence indicate treatment with request. Low values occur in malnutrition associated with hypoproteinaemia. (Approximate reference values: days 0–10, 75–325 nmol/l; children over 1 m, 51–175 nmol/l; values over 126 or less than 54 nmol/l should be reviewed).

Serum tri-iodothyronine (T_3) is only required when initial tests for *hyper*thyroidism are equivocal.

Serum thyroid stimulating hormone (TSH).—Measurement is important, when serum T_4 is low, to confirm *primary* hypothyroidism in which TSH is increased. Levels are normally high over days 0–3 (consult local laboratory for reference values). Basal levels are unreliable in hypothyroidism *secondary* to TSH deficiency when the following test should be used:

Thyroid releasing hormone (TRH) *stimulation test.*—The recumbent patient is given 200 µg of TRH as a single intravenous injection. Serum samples (5 ml to 2 ml minimum) are taken before and 30 and 60 minutes after the injection for TSH assay. A 3–6-fold increase above basal levels can be expected. Patients with hypothalamic disorders of TRH production frequently show higher TSH values after TRH at 60 minutes, when compared with 30-minute samples. Data for euthyroid children is sparse and shows considerable individual variation. Substitution therapy in children should be based on other tests of thyroid function if an impaired response is obtained.

Serum T_3 uptake test.—Not to be confused with T_3 measurements. This should be requested with T_4 measurements when screening for primary hypothyroidism. It indicates thyroxine binding globulin (TBG) sites unoccupied by thyroxine. High values are characteristic of hypothyroidism. Decreased values are found in *hyper*thyroidism. Approximate reference values in children: 54–157.

Renal Function

Water deprivation and pitressin stimulation test.—This gives an early indication of diminished renal tubular efficiency.

Weigh the patient and be prepared to assess clinical dehydration by a further weight, and if necessary discontinue the test. Collect urine and blood for base-line osmolality and/or specific gravity (S.G.) determination. At 18·00 h give the patient a meal and a small amount of fluid not exceeding 150 ml. Prohibit all food and further fluid until the test has been completed.

Collect all further urine samples separately through the night and following morning until the osmolality or S.G. is constant and check that a 5 per cent loss in weight has occurred.

In unimpaired renal function, at least one urine specimen will have an S.G. of 1024 or greater (osmolality over 800 mosmol/kg) and the plasma osmolality will remain normal (275–295 mosmol/kg). In severe renal failure the S.G. may be around 1010 (osmolality less than 300 mosmol/kg) and the plasma osmolality may be greater than normal. In nephrogenic diabetes insipidus the S.G. often is as low as 1001 and the osmolality down to 100 mosmol/kg.

With moderate impairment of renal function the highest urine S.G. and osmolality will be between these values.

If indicated, proceed to pitressin stimulation by taking a further sample of blood and injecting 0·25 units pitressin tannate in oil/10 kg body weight. Continue separate urine collections as passed and collect a further blood sample 2 h after injection. The effect of pitressin on the concentration of these further specimens should be noted. Supplies of pitressin tannate in oil are being discontinued. Synthetic vasopressin (DDAVP) may be a suitable alternative but confident criteria are yet to be established.

Endogenous creatinine clearance.—This gives an assessment of the extent of renal damage and in normal subjects is proportional to glomerular filtration. The height, weight, age and sex of the patient must be notified to the laboratory. The collections of urine must be complete in volume and accurate in timing. Their duration should be determined by the voiding of urine and not by the clock.

Normal activity, diet and fluid intake are encouraged on the day before the test. On the day of the test the child should remain reclining. Breakfast should be light, avoiding meat protein. If it is necessary for the continued co-operation of the patient, milk or a biscuit may be given.

To ensure an adequate flow of urine (approx. 2 ml/min/m²) 10 ml/kg water, flavoured if desired, should be given during the hour before the test. During the test, approx. 09·00–15·00 h, fluid should be given at half this rate, i.e. 5 ml/kg/h, drinks being given at approximately half-hourly intervals.

At about 09·00 h patient empties bladder completely, and the urine is discarded and the time recorded. All urine that is now passed up to approximately 12·00 h is collected and combined as specimen A. The nearest time to 12·00 h of voiding the last specimen is recorded and this ends the first collection.

At about 12·00 h blood (5 ml, plain tube) is taken for analysis and sent straight to the laboratory. All urine passed after the end of the first collection and up to and including a specimen passed at about 15·00 h is collected and combined as specimen B. The time of voiding this last specimen is recorded accurately. This allows two separate calculations of clearance to be made. If these do not agree the test is repeated.

The mean normal value for endogenous creatinine clearances is 123 ($\pm$ 20 per cent) ml/min/1·73 m² body surface area. In very young children, lower values may be normal, e.g. 36 ml/min/1·73 m² at one week.

Special Tests

Galactosaemia.—If on milk, a positive Benedict's (Clinitest) and negative glucose oxidase (Clinistix) is strongly suggestive. Do not exclude the diagnosis on this evidence. Confirm by erythrocyte enzyme assay.

Gangliosidoses.—GM₁–leucocyte β-galactosidase; GM₂–total leucocyte hexosaminidase and separation of isoenzymes A and B to distinguish infantile Tay-Sachs from the Sandhoff variant.

Glycogen storage diseases.—Glucagon test before and after carbohydrate feed (measure both glucose and lactate, (see page 140), glucose during galactose infusion, and erythrocyte glycogen. Liver or leucocyte enzyme assay only for confirmation.

Homocystinuria.—Cyanide-nitroprusside test on urine. Plasma chromatography. Hypermethioninaemia especially in infancy. Treat prior to surgery or during dehydrating illness with pyridoxine 500 mg daily and reduce when the risk of thrombosis lessens.

Lesch-Nyhan syndrome.—Urine uric acid/creatinine ratio. Restrict dietary purine and pass urine directly into laboratory container or send in collecting bags: uric acid precipitates in normal ward container and may be lost.

Lipidaemias.—Plasma cholesterol, triglyceride and lipoprotein electrophoresis after a prolonged (18 h) fast.

Metachromatic leucodystrophy.–Leucocyte arysulphatase A.

Mucopolysaccharidoses.—18–24 h urine collection, kept cold, to avoid false reactions. Alcian Blue (not Toluidine Blue) spot test and bovine albumin (not CPC) turbidity test followed by electrophoresis of urinary MPS for typing.

Organic acidaemias.—Low standard bicarbonate (pH may be normal), gas chromatography of urine (kept frozen).

Phenylketonuria.—Plasma phenylalanine concentration.

Porphyria.—Quantitative urine aminolaevulinic acid (ALA) and porphobilinogen (PBG), copro- and uroporphyrin. Children in remission may require a glycine load before abnormal results can be demonstrated. Faecal porphyrins and erythrocyte protoporphyria.

Suxamethonium sensitivity.—Plasma cholinesterase with and without dibucaine and fluoride inhibition. Urgent analysis is not necessary.

Wilson's disease.—Plasma caeruloplasmin (phenylene diamine oxidase), urinary and plasma copper.

NOTE. Raine, D. N., *Treatment of Inherited Metabolic Disease*, 1975 (M. T. P., Lancaster) gives detailed advice on treating several diseases, and references reporting attempts to treat some 200 others, together with the sources of special dietary preparations throughout the world.

D.N.R.
B.T.R.

GASTRO-INTESTINAL FUNCTION

INVESTIGATION OF MALABSORPTION

Commoner Causes

1. **Persistent post-infective diarrhoea** in young infants is frequently associated with secondary disaccharidase deficiency leading to disaccharide (lactose and possibly sucrose) intolerance. Stools contain fluid which is acid (pH 5·5 or less) and/or positive for reducing substances (see below). Severe cases may also be intolerant of monosaccharides as well.

Specific inborn errors of sugar absorption as a cause of fluid diarrhoea are rare, i.e. specific lactase deficiency, sucrase-isomaltase deficiency, glucose galactose malabsorption (fructose can be absorbed).

2. **Coeliac disease** or permanent gluten intolerance. Minimum diagnostic criteria include evidence of malabsorption (e.g. fat or xylose), abnormal upper small bowel mucosal histology demonstrated by peroral biopsy and good clinical response to gluten-free diet (see page 38). Peroral biopsy is a safe procedure in experienced hands even in small infants, with the exception of those who are very marasmic. However it should be restricted to centres where sufficient experience is constantly gained both to ensure the minimum of technical difficulties for the patient's benefit, and correct interpretation of findings.

3. **Cystic fibrosis.**—Suspected from association of chronic respiratory symptoms with failure to thrive and bulky stools with an offensive *penetrating* odour.

The sweat test is the most definitive test and the presence of *fat globules in stool* is simple and of especial value in infants with suggestive respiratory symptoms (see below).

Approximately 90 per cent of C.F. patients have pancreatic insufficiency and therefore steatorrhoea. Examination of stools for fat globules is usually sufficient to demonstrate this and fat balance or duodenal intubation is only necessary in doubtful cases.

DETAILS OF TESTS

Stool microscopy—Cysts and ova indicate infestation with protozoa (giardia lamblia) or worms. Giardial infestation may be present even in absence of cysts in stool—motile forms can be seen in warm duodenal fluid or on villous surface mucosal biopsies.

Fat globules result from defective intraluminal digestion either from pancreatic insufficiency or biliary obstruction. Place on microscope slide small portion faeces + drop of water—mix together with glass rod—add coverslip and examine under microscope. In patients with pancreatic insufficiency numerous yellow shiny spherical globules of varied size will be seen in each field, either low or high power. Differentiate from air bubbles (colourless), starch grains (oval). The presence of undigested vegetable matter is not important.

Stool pH.—Test *fluid* part of stool with pH indicator paper —pH 5·5 or less is abnormal and usually indicates sugar malabsorption (colonic bacteria ferment sugars to lactic acid).

Reducing substances in stool.—Use freshly passed stool and examine fluid part (collection will require plastic napkin liner or other manoeuvre). Mix 2 vol. water to 1 vol. faeces. Place 15 drops of mixture in tube and add 1 Clinitest tablet. Read colour on Clinitest chart. Quarter per cent or less is negative; $\frac{1}{4}$–$\frac{1}{2}$ per cent suspect; $\frac{1}{2}$ per cent or more is positive for reducing sugar (e.g. lactose or monosaccharides, glucose, galactose or fructose) and suggests sugar intolerance. For demonstration of sucrose dilute HCl should be added to stool mixture which is then boiled before Clinitest tablet is added.

Faecal fat excretion (quantitative).—Collect all stools for three consecutive days. If stools are passed irregularly and days are missed, the collection should be extended for a fourth or fifth day. In children over 6 months of age a normal average daily excretion on an adequate intake of fat for age should not exceed 14 mmol (4 g) per day. It is not necessary to measure the intake of fat accurately but an estimate should be made using food tables of the fat in the diet which in young children comes from milk (volume taken), butter, eggs, cheese.

Raised fat excretion is a reliable index of malabsorption but does not differentiate underlying pathology.

Urinary xylose excretion method.—Having fasted from the previous evening, the patient should empty his bladder at 07·30 h, the urine being discarded. 5 g of D-xylose in 100 ml of water is then given and followed during the next hour by 150 ml of water when desired by the patient. Urine is collected for five hours after the xylose. Normally, at least 25 per cent (1 g) of the dose is recoverable in the urine. Test is often unreliable in young children because of collection difficulties.

One hour blood xylose method (infants and children under 30 kg).—Following a fast of at least 6 hours, the patient is given 5 g of D-xylose, in 100 ml of water, Exactly 1 hour later, 1–2 ml of venous blood is taken into a standard fluoride (blood sugar) tube. A one hour blood level above 1·3 mmol/l (20 mg/100 ml) is normal. A result below this is abnormal but should be confirmed by a repeat test the next day.

The one hour blood xylose level indicates rate of absorption in the upper gut and is abnormal when the mucosal brush border is damaged.

Sweat test using pilocarpine iontophoresis. Na and Cl levels above 60 mmol/l denote cystic fibrosis provided at least 100 mg of sweat is obtained and the difference between Na and Cl is less than 30 mmol/l. If the individual values lie between 45 and 75 the test should be repeated. It is reliable from the age of three weeks; small infants should be well wrapped and two gauze swabs used simultaneously.

M.J.B.

X

MISCELLANEOUS

MANAGEMENT OF CHILDREN WITH NON-ACCIDENTAL INJURIES ("BATTERED BABY" SYNDROME)

THE diagnosis of child abuse is often missed, and trauma inflicted by the parents must be considered in any case where symptoms remain unexplained. These children often present to the Casualty Department, and the diagnosis should be suspected in any young child presenting with bruising, particularly of the face, and/or with underlying fractures.

Diagnosis

History.—Suspicion should be aroused when:

(a) There has been delay in taking the child to a doctor.

(b) There is inadequate, discrepant or excessively plausible explanation of the injury.

(c) The child or a sibling has previously attended hospital with an injury, or when a history of previous injury is obtained.

(d) There is evidence of repeated injury.

(e) The child is frequently brought to the doctor or hospital for little apparent reason.

(f) Parents exhibit disturbed behaviour or unusual reaction to the child's injuries.

(g) The child fails to thrive or shows obvious neglect.

Examination.—At first sight the injuries may appear trivial, for example: small facial bruises, burns or abrasions; injuries to the mouth; injuries caused by severe shaking, e.g. bruising from handling. A full examination of the child is essential to detect any other new or old injuries, followed by a skeletal survey.

Immediate Management

If the diagnosis seems at all possible:

1. *Admit the child* to hospital. This should be done whether or not the actual medical and surgical findings are severe enough to warrant admission. Admission offers an opportunity to assess and protect the child.

153

2. *Skeletal survey* (X-ray of long bones, ribs and skull) is essential, and consultation with the radiologist will be most helpful in estimating the date of any fractures.
3. *Record carefully* the history and clinical findings with diagrams.
4. *Exclude a bleeding disorder* both for medical and legal reasons.
5. *Photographs* (black and white or coloured) are helpful in documenting findings.
6. *No accusations should be made against the parents* as this antagonises them and makes further management complicated.
7. *Refer the parents to a Medical Social Worker* for further family investigation.
8. *The paediatrician-in-charge should make the decision about involving the police or social services:* when a Medical Social Worker is involved this will be in consultation.

Subsequent Management

Discussion with the parents should be the responsibility of an experienced paediatrician. He will assess the mental status of the parents and make recommendations on the subsequent management of the family. Although every effort will be made to maintain the family unit the child's safety is the aim of management. It may be necessary to bring the child before the Juvenile Court so that on discharge from hospital its safety may be guaranteed.

The house physician may be confronted by an irate parent demanding the discharge of his child. Every effort should be made to placate such parents and to explain that the child's medical condition is still under investigation. If despite such effort the parents insist on discharge, the action recommended is:

1. Contact the registrar or consultant in charge of the case and inform them that the parents are insisting on discharging their child against medical advice.
2. If the consultant feels that it is not in the child's interests to be discharged at the present time, the Social Services Department should be contacted. An application will be made by this department to the Justice of the Peace who can order that the child remains in hospital.

3. If for any reason there is a delay or difficulty in obtaining a safety order, the Police Department should be contacted by a member of the medical staff.

NUCLEAR SEXING AND CHROMOSOMAL ANALYSIS

Nuclear sexing is a cheap and accurate first step towards the elucidation of ambiguous sex, mental retardation and dwarfism. Sex chromatin (inactivated X chromosome) and the Y chromosome are recognisable with appropriate stains. The results are often more important than chromosomal analysis alone. If the nuclear sexing results are inappropriate for sex, then chromosomal analysis should follow.

The Indications for Chromosomal Analysis

(a) Inappropriate nuclear sexing result: e.g. chromatin–ve girl.

(b) Unexplained mental retardation (particularly if associated with malformation such as cleft palate, coloboma of eye, congenital heart defect, deformity of ears, defects of hands and feet).

(c) Infants suspected of having trisomy 21, 18, or 13.*

(d) Other newborn infants with multiple defects [as listed in (b)].

GENETIC COUNSELLING

The recurrence risk of disorders will frequently be of interest to parents; when it is very low, as is usual in mongolism or

*Most correctly diagnosed cases have an extra free-lying chromosome. In a few infants the extra chromosome material is found to be translocated onto another chromosome; in such cases the chromosomes of both parents must always be analysed. As these are often normal it must be assumed that the translocation was a recent and isolated event and therefore unlikely to recur, but sometimes one or other parent has a balanced arrangement and therefore runs the risk of having further affected infants. For example 6 per cent of mongols have a 21 translocation but only a third of these have a parent with a balanced translocation. Trisomy 21 may recur in a sibship if the mother is a mongol or mongol mosaic (trisomy 21/normal). A number of apparently normal mothers have been discovered with this form of mosaicism which can only be excluded by careful chromosomal analysis. The incidence of trisomy 21 depends on maternal age. Below 30 years the risk is 1–2000. At about 35 years the incidence rises steeply to become 1–50 at 45 years.

most rare malformations, or very high, as in fibrocystic disease, the parents should normally be informed.

Simple genetic disorders in man are due either to mutations which may be recent and unlikely to recur in sibs (i.e. in mongolism, or in dominant disorders born to normal parents) or they may be due to some distant mutation as in almost all cases of autosomal recessive disorders (e.g. albinism, fibrocystic disease) and many cases of sex-linked disorder (e.g. haemophilia, Duchenne's dystrophy).

In congenital malformations, as in all diseases, there is a familial tendency but this is usually too small to influence further conceptions. In almost all malformations the aetiology is unknown and the empiric recurrence risk is 3 to 5 per cent, and about 10 per cent after two affected children.

In recessively determined disorders in which the diagnosis is accurate, and legitimacy can be assumed, the recurrence risk is 25 per cent. The commonest forms include fibrocystic disease, albinism, the adrenogenital syndrome, and haemoglobino-pathies.

In sex-linked disorders, such as haemophilia and Duchenne's muscular dystrophy, isolated cases may be due to either new or old mutants and there may, or may not, be increased risk.

Dominant conditions, such as the common form of achondroplasia, are rare and, if the parents are free of disease and the diagnosis accurate, it may be assumed that this is due to a new mutation carrying no realistic risk of recurrence.

AMNIOCENTESIS

Selective abortion is feasible when the diagnosis can be made from the examination of supernatant amniotic fluid or by examining amniotic fluid cells in cases where the defect is expressed in these cells.

At present alpha-fetoprotein is the main constituent routinely sought in supernatant fluid. The level is raised whenever the protein has the opportunity to leak out from the fetus as in open neural tube defects, some cases of exomphalos, congenital nephrosis and fetal death. Cells can be examined for nuclear sex bodies, chromosomes and certain rare and specific metabolic disorders.

The main indications for sixteen-week amniocentesis are:

Chromosomal
1. When a parent has a balanced translocation or re-arrangement.
2. Mother has had a previous trisomic mongol.
3. Maternal age over 40 years.

Alpha-fetoprotein (for open neural tube defect)
1. Previous neural tube defect baby.
2. Parental spina bifida.

Sex chromatin
1. X-linked disease if mother probably a carrier or if father affected when all daughters would be carriers.

Metabolic disease

Few laboratories are competent to culture and test for those rare metabolic disorders amenable to antenatal diagnosis. Clinical genetics and paediatric biochemical departments hold current lists of laboratories willing to advise on and undertake these tests.

Most main cytogenetic laboratories can undertake nuclear sexing by examination for sex chromatin and Y chromosome fluorescence and undertake chromosomal analysis. Few biochemical laboratories can provide a diagnostic service for their metabolic problems. Clinical geneticists and paediatric biochemists in the U.K. hold current lists of disorders amenable to diagnosis and of laboratories competent to carry out the analyses. It is usually recommended that only centres with ultrasound facilities should undertake amniocentesis as twinning provides problems and maturity has to be confirmed.

FITS IN CHILDHOOD

The treatment of fits in childhood may be grouped as follows:

1. *Neonatal fits.*—These are often symptomatic of a treatable condition (see page 67). Infants usually tolerate phenobarbitone well. Diazepam may be used.
2. *Infantile spasms* (West syndrome) initially respond best to corticosteroids or ACTH, but nitrazepam, clonazepam, or sodium valproate can then be used to maintain control of the epilepsy.

3. *Febrile convulsions.*—The arguments over therapy persist; continuous phenobarbitone may help up to the age of 18 months, but phenobarbitone or phenytoin given at the time of fever are of no value. Sodium valproate at the time of the first convulsion may prevent a second convulsion. Intravenous diazepam is the therapy of choice but intramuscular paraldehyde is safer in an outpatient.

4. *Myoclonic astatic epilepsy* (Lennox syndrome) may respond temporarily to corticosteroids or ACTH, but the drugs of choice for maintenance therapy are sodium valproate, nitrazepam and clonazepam. Other myoclonic epilepsies, including those with photosensitivity, respond best to sodium valproate.

5. *Absences* with 3 c/s spike and wave (petit mal) respond best to sodium valproate, though many will respond to ethosuximide. Absences with automatisms often do not respond to ethosuximide alone but nearly always respond to sodium valproate.

6. *Tonic clonic seizures* (grand mal) in children are best treated with sodium valproate because this drug does not sedate, or produce undesirable effects. It often makes patients more lively and alert. Phenytoin can be used, but is undesirable particularly in females because of its side-effects. If phenytoin is used *accurate* serum levels are essential.

7. *Focal fits* (motor or sensory) respond best to carbamazepine but can be treated with primidone or phenobarbitone or phenytoin.

8. *Temporal lobe epilepsy* is best treated with carbamazepine alone. If phenytoin is used in males effective therapy depends on accurate serum levels and cannot be assessed on the basis of mg/kg.

Since the half-life of many anticonvulsants exceeds 12 hours, most can be given once or twice a day after the patient has been stabilised. Phenobarbitone, primidone, phenytoin, ethosuximide can all be given once a day. Carbamazepine and sodium valproate should be given twice a day, but occasionally an afternoon dose is needed.

Few anti-epileptic drugs act rapidly, many take a week or more to reach a steady level, and may not achieve the full effect for a month. The Table summarises the peak time, steady level time, effective serum level, half life and usual maintenance dosage. For side-effects see p. 88 *B.N.F.*, 1976.

ANTICONVULSANTS

	Peak single dose	Steady level	Effective serum level μg/ml	Half-life hours	Usual maintenance dosage for children
Phenobarbitone	6–18 h	7 d	15–25	37–73	30–60 mg once daily
Phenytoin	5 h	7 d	10–20	22	50–150 mg once daily
Carbamazepine	6–12 h	32 h	6–8	17	200–400 mg twice daily
Nitrazepam	2 h	—	—	24	2·5–10 mg nightly
Ethosuximide	1–4 h	7 + d	40–80	30	250–500 mg once daily
Sodium valproate	1½ h	—	60–80	8–15	300–900 mg twice daily

REPORTING DEATHS TO THE CORONER

In deaths in the following circumstances the doctor is advised to inform the coroner as soon as possible:

All Deaths which are sudden or unexpected and where the Doctor cannot certify the real, as opposed to the terminal, cause of death or where the Doctor has not attended in the last illness or within fourteen days of death.

Abortions—other than natural.

Accidents and Injuries of any date, if in any way contributing to the cause of death.

Alcoholism—chronic or acute.

Anaesthetics and Operations—deaths while under the influence of anaesthetics and deaths following operation for injury or where the operation, however necessarily or skilfully performed, may have precipitated or expedited death.

Crime or Suspected Crime.

Drugs—therapeutic mishaps, abuse or addiction.

Ill-Treatment—starvation or neglect.

Industrial Diseases arising out of the deceased's employment, e.g. pneumoconiosis, Weil's disease and all diseases and poisons covered by the Factories Acts.

Infant Deaths—if in any way obscure.

Pensioners receiving Disability Pensions. Where death might be connected with the pensionable disability.

Persons in Legal Custody—in a Prison, Borstal Institution or Approved School, or any Detention Quarters even if the death was in hospital.

Persons suffering from mental disorders are to be reported only if they fall into one of the general categories.

Poisoning from any cause, occupational, therapeutic, accidental, suicidal, homicidal; also food poisoning.

Septicaemias—if originating from an injury or an operation.

Stillbirths—where there may be a possibility of the child having been born alive, or where there is suspicion.

N.B. A provisionally registered practitioner can only sign a death certificate in the course of his duties at an approved institution.

Cremation Certificate Form C can only be signed by a practitioner who has been fully registered for more than five years (any period of provisional registration does not qualify).

Apart from the general rule of law some Coroners have special wishes such as requesting that deaths within 24 hours of admission should be reported to him.

Sudden infant death syndrome (cot deaths) would automatically be reported and any case where there has been recent or possibly relevant injury should also be reported. The reasons for this are not bureaucratic formality but to avoid inconvenience and distress to relatives if the death certificate is questioned at the Registrar's office and possibly reported to the Coroner at this stage. If in doubt therefore it is best to ring the Coroner's Officer and this will smooth the passage of the certificate and does not necessarily result in a post-mortem.

Advice on Attending an Inquest

First, it is important to attend the post-mortem with all the relevant clinical notes and X-rays. If required to attend the inquest, the doctor should be punctual, bring the relevant documents and refresh his memory from the notes and statements on the evidence especially regarding dates, times and special procedures. The medical evidence will help to achieve the objects of an inquest which are:

1. To ascertain on behalf of the Crown whether any criminal act was relevant, but equally important are the following:
2. To bring out all the evidence about what happened so that the relatives will have as complete a picture as possible as to how death occurred; this may prevent subsequent criticism of medical treatment given.
3. To try and see if anything can be learnt or done with a view to preventing similar tragedies.
4. To reach a verdict.

[NOTES]

[NOTES]

[NOTES]

XI

PAEDIATRIC PRESCRIBING

ALL prescriptions should be clearly written using English or approved abbreviations. The use of vague terms like S.O.S. and P.R.N. is to be deprecated.

In general, single drugs should be prescribed always using approved names and metric doses. In prescription writing "g" is the international abbreviation for gramme and for amounts less than 0·1 g mg should be written. Quantities less than 1 mg should be given in micrograms. The *B.N.F.* 1976–78 states "The accepted symbol for microgram is "μg". On prescriptions "microgram" should always be written in full; elsewhere where an abbreviation is essential "mcg" may be used.

For oral liquid preparations wherever possible the dose is supplied in a 5 ml volume and the patient issued with a 5 ml spoon. However, reasons of stability and palatability sometimes dictate other dose volumes; it is better for the prescriber to order the required dose, leaving the volume to the pharmacist.

The labels of all dispensed preparations should bear full details of content unless otherwise requested.

Prescriptions for Controlled Drugs [e.g. Morphine, Pethidine Cocaine, Phenoperidine and their derivatives; Amphetamine, Dexamphetamine, Methylphenidate, Phenmetrazine, Methaqualone (including 'Mandrax')] must state dose, total number of doses written in both figures and letters, frequency of administration of the drug, bear the full signature (initials are not sufficient) of a registered Medical/Dental Practitioner and finally the date.

CALCULATION OF DOSAGE FOR CHILDREN

Many methods have been suggested for determining the size of paediatric doses, but there is general agreement that calculations based on body surface area provide the most reliable estimate of therapeutic dose. A nomogram calculation of surface area from the height and weight of the infant is shown on page 168.

Since body surface area is not easily determined and doses/m^2 are not easily remembered, the surface area and hence the

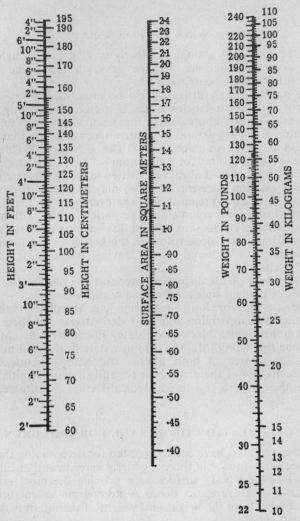

Surface area nomogram. (Adapted from J. R. Geigy, S.A., data.)

dose has been expressed as a percentage of the adult (after Catzel).*

The following table adapted from Catzel's percentage method correlates both age and weight assuming that the child is of average size but does not apply to the newborn.

Age	Average Weight in		Dose as Percentage of Adult Dose	In mg/kg if Adult Dose = 1·0 mg/kg
	kg	lb		
Over 2 weeks ..	3·2	7	12 ⎫	2·0
4 months ..	6·5	14	20 ⎭	
1 year	10·0	22	25 ⎫	
3 years	15·0	33	33 ⎬	1·5
7 years	23	51	50 ⎭	
12 years	37	82	75	1·25
Adult	66	145	100	1·0

Drugs having a wide therapeutic index can be dealt with on an age basis but where the range between the therapeutic and the toxic level is narrow or where intensive therapy is needed in an ill child, the dose must be tailored more accurately to the individual weight. For a fat child the dose for age rather than weight should be used, fat playing little part in drug metabolism. In the dosage tables that follow, these principles have been followed except that the dose for the child aged one year and under has been shown on a uniform mg/kg basis, which results in slight underdosage for the first few months of life. This should be borne in mind if high blood levels are needed for a particular situation or when a new drug is being used. The above table can then be applied after consulting the literature concerning the specific product.

All Doses stated are Single Doses

Where a drug needs to be repeated several times daily to give a therapeutic blood level, the recommended number of times per 24 hours is given in column three.

* Catzel, P. (1974). *Paediatric Prescriber*, 4th edit. Oxford: Blackwell Scientific Publications.

Once the dose has been calculated, prescribers are asked to refer to the last column in the dosage section as a guide to a measurable dose. e.g. Chlorothiazide for a 12 year old = 700 mg. The nearest measurable dose would be 750 mg, i.e. 1½ 500 mg tablets.

N.B. A dash (viz.—) in a dosage column indicates that the drug is not normally given in this age group.

Intrathecal Doses

Paediatric doses have been estimated by reducing the adult dose to 75 per cent at 12, 50 per cent at 7. The dose should not be less than 25 per cent of the adult dose at any age.

Proprietary Names

Proprietary names are omitted; if necessary refer to page 328 *B.N.F.* 1976–78.

SOME IMPORTANT DRUGS

Drug	Route	Times Daily	DOSE Caution. Read calculation of dosage for children on page 167						Availability and Remarks
			0-2/52 Neonatal	2/52- 1 year	1 year	7 years	Adult		
Acetazolamide	Oral	Once	—	—	125 mg	250 mg	500 mg		Tab. 250 mg scored. Sustets 500 mg Twice daily for Glaucoma
Adrenaline inj. 1-1000	S.C.	Single dose	—	0·01ml/kg	0·12 ml	0·25 ml	0·5 ml		For treatment of status asthmaticus see page 93
Allopurinol	Oral	3	—	5 mg/kg	50 mg	100 mg	200 mg		Prevention of uric acid nephropathy. N.B. Potentiates 6-Mercaptopurine— reduce 6MP dose by 75%. See page 126. Tabs. 100 mg.
Aluminium hydroxide mixture B.P.C.	Oral	3 or 4	—	—	1 ml	2·5 ml	5 ml		
Aminocaproic Acid (E.A.C.A.)	Oral I.V.	4	—	100 mg/kg	1·5 g	3 g	6 g		Eff. Powder, Syrup, and Inj. Management of oral bleeding in coagulation disorders. I.V. dose by infusion (not bolus) 6-hourly.
Aminophylline	I.M. I.V.	3 or 4	—		40 mg	80 mg	250-500 mg		I.M. painful, see Diprophylline. I.V. 250 mg/10 ml inj. very slowly or by infusion. Suppos. for newborn see page 67.
Amitriptyline HCl	Oral	3	—	—	—	10 mg	25 mg		Antidepressant dose which may be doubled. Nocturnal enuresis dose. Tabs. 10 mg, 25 mg and Syrup.
					10 mg to 25 mg at night				
Amodiaquine	Oral	3	—	5 mg/kg	50 mg	100 mg	200 mg		1st day give stated dose 8-hourly, then daily for 4 days. Tabs. 200 mg.

SOME IMPORTANT DRUGS—(Continued)

Drug	Route	Times Daily	0-2/52 Neonatal	2/52-1 year	1 year	7 years	Adult	Availability and Remarks
								DOSE Caution. Read calculation of dosage for children on page 167
Amylobarbitone and Sodium salt	Oral I.M. I.V.	3 or 4	5 mg/kg		50 mg	100 mg	200 mg	Hypnotic dose. May be increased in Status Epilepticus. Amylobarb. Tabs. 15, 30, 50 mg. Amylobarb. Sod. Tabs. 60, 200 mg.
Asparaginase	I.V.		For Leukaemia see page 126.					Warning: may cause anaphylaxis
Aspirin and Soluble Aspirin	Oral	3 or 4	Suggest Paracetamol			300 mg	600 mg	Tabs. and Soluble Tabs. 300 mg. Up to 100 mg/kg/day for Rheumatic Fever. Adjust to Salicylate level.
Atropine methonitrate	Oral	Before feeds	50 mcg/kg		500 mcg	—	—	"Eumydrin". Drops only.
Atropine sulphate	Oral or S.C.	Single	15 mcg/kg		150 mcg	300 mcg	600 mcg	Tabs. 400 mcg and 600 mcg. Pre-op. dose.
Bendrofluazide	Oral	Once	1·25 mg		1·25 mg	2·5 mg	5 mg	K^+ supplements required. Tabs. 2·5 mg, 5 mg.
Benorylate	Oral	4	—	25 mg/kg	250 mg	500 mg –1 g	2 g	Tab. 750 mg. Susp. For Rheumatoid arthritis.
Bephenium hydroxynaphthoate	Oral	Once	—	2·5 g			5 g	Sachets 5 g. Hookworms (Ancylostomiasis) and Roundworms (Ascariasis).
Bethanidine sulphate	Oral	Twice	—		2·5 mg	5 mg	10 mg	Initial dose stated. Increase according to response up to 20 × initial dose. Severe hypertension, see page 99. Tabs. 10 mg, 50 mg.
Bromhexine	Oral	4	—		4 mg b.d.	4 mg	8 mg	Tabs. 8 mg. Syrup.

	Route	Freq.		3000 units to 5000 units			
Calciferol (Vit. D₂)	Oral	Once		3000 units to 5000 units			Calciferol-sensitive rickets dose. Tabs. 3000 and 50,000 units.
Calcium chloride as dihydrate	Oral	4	33 mg/kg	330 mg	—	—	See page 49. 5 ml Inj. CaCl₂ . 2H₂O contains 2·5 mmol Ca⁺⁺ ≡ 100 mg Ca⁺⁺ (0·45 ml ≡ 33 mg CaCl₂ . 2H₂O).
Calcium gluconate	Oral	4	100 mg/kg	1 g	2 g	4 g	1 g = 2·25 mmol Ca⁺⁺ = 90 mg Ca⁺⁺. See page 49. Tabs. 300 mg and 600 mg Syrup.
	I.V.	Single	30 mg/kg Slow I.V. using 10% Inj. diluted to 2·5% solution.				Effervescent Tabs. 1 g. Caution—Bradycardia.
Calcium lactate	Oral	4	75 mg/kg	750 mg	1·5 g	3 g	1 g = 3·25 mmol Ca⁺⁺ = 130 mg Ca⁺⁺. Tabs. 330 mg.
Carbachol	S.C.	4	6 mcg/kg	60 mcg	125 mcg	250 mcg	Oral dose 4 times S.C. Scored tabs. 2 mg.
Carbamazepine	Oral	2 or 3	10 mg/kg	100 mg	200 mg	400 mg	Grand Mal Epilepsy dose. Tabs. 100 mg and 200 mg.
Carbimazole	Oral	3	0·25 mg/kg	2·5 mg	5 mg	10 mg	Initial dose stated. Reduce total daily dose to 1/3 or 1/4 when symptoms controlled and give as single daily dose. Tabs. 5 mg.
Chloral hydrate	Oral	3	30 mg/kg	300 mg	600 mg at night	1·5 g at night	Single hypnotic dose can be doubled.
Chlorothiazide	Oral	Once	125 mg	250 mg	500 mg	1 g	Scored Tabs. 500 mg. K⁺ supplement required. Prems. only 62·5 mg dose.
Chloroquine as base	Oral	Once	7·5 mg/kg	75 mg	150 mg	300 mg	Tab. Chlor. Phos. 250 mg = 150 mg base. Tab. Chlor. Sulph. 200mg = 150 mg base. Syrup 50 mg base in 5 ml. Follow with Primaquine for 14 days. Amoebiasis—up to twice stated dose.
			In acute malaria initially TWICE stated dose, then stated dose 6 hrs later and daily for 2 days.				
	I.V.		5 mg/kg in 150 ml. Inj. Sod. Chlor. 0·9% slowly. Repeat in 12 hours.				Inj. Chlor. Sulph. contains 40 mg base in 1 ml.
	I.M.	Once	5 mg/kg for 5 days				Caution in children.

SOME IMPORTANT DRUGS—(Continued)

Drug	Route	Times Daily	DOSE. Caution. Read calculation of dosage for children on page 167					Availability and Remarks
			0-2/52 Neonatal	2/52-1 year	1 year	7 years	Adult	
Chlorpheniramine	Oral	3 or 4	—	—	1 mg	2 mg	4 mg	Dose may be safely doubled. Tabs. 4 mg, 8 mg and 12 mg (long-acting) and Syrup.
	S.C. or I.V.	Single	—	0.25 mg/kg	2.5 mg	5 mg	10 mg	
Chlorpromazine	Oral or I.M.	3 or 4	—	1 mg/kg	10 mg	25 mg	50 mg	Sedative/Antiemetic dose stated. Psychiatric dose—stated dose × 2. Neonatal tetanus 2-4 mg/kg. Tabs. 10 mg, 25 mg, 50 mg, and 100 mg. Syrup.
Choline theophyllinate	Oral	3	—	5 mg/kg	50 mg	100 mg	200 mg	Tabs. 100 and 200 mg. Syrup. Double dose in severe asthma with monitoring.
Clonazepam	Oral maint.	3 or 4	—	—	0.5 mg	1 mg	2 mg	Tab. 0.5 mg and 2 mg. May cause drowsiness, start with lower doses inc. to maint.
Codeine linctus B.P.C.	Oral	3 or 4	—	—	1.25 ml	2.5 ml	5 ml	
Cyclizine	Oral or I.M.	3	—	1 mg/kg	12.5 mg	25 mg	50 mg	Scored Tabs. 50 mg.
Cyclophosphamide	Oral or I.V.	Once	3 mg/kg		50 mg	100 mg	200 mg	I.V. therapy for 5 days used initially for neoplasms. Initial oral dose stated (nephrotic syndrome and neoplastic disease) adjust dose on W.C. Count. For leukaemia see page 126. Tabs. 10 mg, 50 mg.
Cytosine Arabinoside	I.V. S.C.	Once	For use in Leukaemia see page 126.					For I/T do NOT use special diluent.

Drug	Route	Frequency						Remarks
Daunorubicin	I.V.	Once	For use in Leukaemia see page 126.					Total cumulative dose not to exceed 350 mg/m² because of cardiotoxicity.
Desferrioxamine mesylate		Once	80 mg/kg I.V. in 24 hours at rate of not more than 15 mg/hour.					Iron poisoning see page 116.
Desmopressin (DDAVP)	Nasal	1 or 2	—		5–10 mcg		10–20 mcg	Nasal soln. 100 mcg/ml. For diabetes insipidus, replaces Pitressin Tannate in Oil.
Diazepam	Oral I.M. I.V.	4	0.05 mg/kg		0.5 mg	1 mg	2 mg	Mild tranquillising dose.
			0.25 mg/kg		2.5 mg	5 mg	10 mg	Spasmolytic/severe anxiety/anticonvulsant/pre-med. dose. Tabs. 2 mg, 5 mg, 10 mg, Syrup 2 mg/5 ml.
Diazoxide	Oral	2 or 3	5–20 mg/kg/day				100 mg	Coated Tabs. 50 mg. Dose for hypoglycaemia.
	I.V. only	up to 4			5 mg/kg		300 mg	Antihypertensive dose.
Dichloralphenazone	Oral	Once	30 mg/kg		325 mg	650 mg	1–3 g	Tabs. 650 mg, Syrup.
Dicyclomine	Oral	3 or 4	—	0.5 mg/kg	5 mg	10 mg	20 mg	Tabs. 10 mg. Syrup.
Digoxin	Oral	2	see page 105.				250 mcg	Elixir 50 mcg in 1 ml. Tabs. 62.5 mcg, 125 mcg and 250 mcg.
Dihydrocodeine Bitartrate	Oral	3 or 4	not recommended under 7 years		500 mcg/kg		30–60 mg	Tabs. 30 mg. Syrup. Analgesic dose.
	I.M.	as required	not recommended under 7 years		500 mcg/kg		50 mg	
Dioctyl sodium sulphosuccinate	Oral	3	—		5 mg	10 mg	20 mg	As enema 1 mg/kg. Tabs. 20 mg. Syrup.
Diprophylline	Oral I.M. or I.V.	3	—	5 mg/kg	50 mg	100 mg	200 mg	Tabs. 200 mg. Syrup. Supps. 400 mg and 150 mg.
Droperidol	I.V. I.M. Oral	Once	0.3 mg/kg		3.75 mg	7.5 mg	15 mg	Produces "detachment" pre-neuro-surgery. Normal premedication dose. Tabs. 2.5 mg, 10 mg.
			0.1 mg/kg		1.25 mg	2.5 mg	5 mg	

SOME IMPORTANT DRUGS—(Continued)

Drug	Route	Times Daily	DOSE Caution. Read calculation of dosage for children on page 167					Availability and Remarks
			0-2/52 Neonatal	2/52-1 year	1 year	7 years	Adult	
Edrophonium	I.M.	Single	0·25 mg/kg		2·5 mg	5 mg	10 mg	Test for myasthenia gravis I.V.—give 1/5 dose initially. Remainder slowly if tolerated.
Inj. Emetine HCl.	I.M. S.C.	Once	—	1·5 mg/kg	15 mg	30 mg	60 mg	Acute amoebiasis, Monitor with E.C.G. (myocarditis). See page 80.
Ephedrine	Oral	3	—	0·8 mg/kg	7·5 mg	15 mg	30 mg	Tabs. 30, 15 and 7·5 mg. Elixir B.P.C. 15 mg/5 ml.
Ethacrynic acid	Oral	Once	2·5 mg/kg		25 mg	50 mg	100 mg	Tabs. 50 mg.
Ethosuximide	Oral	Once	—	—	125 mg	250 mg	500 mg	Caps. 250 mg. Syrup. See page 159.
Ferrous sulphate	Oral	3	—	6 mg/kg	60 mg	120 mg	200 mg	Tab. Ferr. Sulph. Co = 200 mg. Paed. Mixt. BNF = 60 mg/5 ml = 12 mg Fe++ = 0·2 mmol Fe++.
Folic acid	Oral	Once	—	250 mcg/kg	2·5 mg	5 mg	10 mg	Tabs. 100 mcg, 500 mcg and 5 mg.
Frusemide	Oral	Alt. days or once daily	1-4 mg/kg/day		20 mg	40 mg	80 mg	Action complete in 3-4 hours. Tabs. 20 mg. Scored tabs. 40 mg. Susp. unstable. I.M. give half oral dose. I.V. give quarter oral dose.
Glucagon	I.M. I.V.	Once	20 mcg/kg		250 mcg	500 mcg	1 mg	Hypoglycaemia. Diagnostic test in glycogen storage disease.
Haloperidol	Oral I.M.	Twice	—	25 mcg/kg	200 mcg	400 mcg	1 mg 5 mg	Liquid 2 mg/ml. Tabs. 1·5 mg. Caps. 0·5 mg.

	Route	Frequency	150 units/kg	2500 units	5000 units	10,000 units	
Heparin	I.V.	—					Repeat 4–6 hourly by continuous infusion as maintenance to maintain the thrombin time or whole-blood clotting time at 2–4 × the control value. Antidote—Protamine Sulphate.
Hydrallazine	Oral / I.M.	4 / 4	— / —	From 1 yr, 0.2 mg/kg Max. 200 mg/day			Tab. 25 mg, 50 mg. Unstable in liquid. For hypertensive crises.
Hyoscine hydrobromide	Oral or S.C.	Single	15 mcg/kg	150 mcg	300 mcg	600 mcg	Premedication dose.
Imipramine	Oral	3 ONCE at night	— / —	— / —	10 mg / 25 mg	25 mg / 50 mg	Antidepressant dose—may be doubled. Nocturnal enuresis. Tabs. 10 mg, 25 mg. Syrup.
Indomethacin	Oral / Rectal	—	— / —	— / 25 mg	25 mg b.d. / 50 mg	25 mg t.d.s. / 100 mg	Caps. 25 mg. Susp. / Supps. 100 mg.
Ipecacuanha	Oral	Single	—	0–12 mths. 5 ml. 1–2 yrs. 10 ml. Over 2 yrs. 15 ml.			Ipecacuanha Paed. Emetic Draught BPC. See BNF page 270.
Ketamine	I.V. / I.M.	Single / ,,	— / —	2 mg/kg 8–12 mg/kg			Must use a sialogogue. Do not disturb during recovery.
Levallorphan tartrate	I.M. or I.V.	Single	Full-term infants 0.25 mg (0.25 ml of 0.1% solution).				See newborn section, page 59.
Magnesium chloride MgCl₂,6H₂O	Oral I.M. I.V.	3 or 4 Once	0.15 mmol/kg (30 mg/kg) in neonatal hypomagnesaemia according to response.				Give I.V. slowly.
Magnesium sulphate MgSO₄.7H₂O	I.M. I.V.	Once	0.15 mmol/kg (0.075 ml/kg 50% Inj.) in neonatal hypomagnesaemia according to response.				Give I.V. slowly.
Mebendazole	Oral	2	—	100 mg 2 years to adults			Tab. 100 mg Anti-helminthic. 3-day course.
Mepacrine HCl.	Oral	Twice	—	25 mg	50 mg	100 mg	Dose for Giardiasis. 5 day course. Tabs. 100 mg.

SOME IMPORTANT DRUGS—(Continued)

Drug	Route	Times Daily	DOSE — Caution. Read calculation of dosage for children on page 167					Availability and Remarks
			0-2/52 Neonatal	2/52-1 year	1 year	7 years	Adult	
Mercaptopurine	Oral							50 mg Tabs. scored.
Methotrexate	Oral		For leukaemia see page 126.					Tabs. 2·5 mg.
Methylcellulose	Oral	Twice	—	—	500 mg	1 g	2 g	Granules 2 g = 1 level 5 ml tsp. Tabs. 500 mg. Both followed by water.
Methyldopa	Oral	3	—	6 mg/kg	62·5 mg	125 mg	250 mg	Increase according to response. Not exceeding 4 times initial dose. Tabs 125 mg, 250 mg, 500 mg.
	I.V.	4	—	6 mg/kg	62·5 mg	125 mg	250 mg	
			Added to 100 ml 50 g/l dextrose and given over 30 minutes.					
Methylphenidate HCl	Oral	2	—	—	1·25 mg	2·5 mg	5 mg	For hyperkinesia. Adjust dose according to response. Tabs. 10 mg.
Metoclopramide	Oral	3	—	0·1 mg/kg	1 mg	5 mg	10 mg	Tabs., 5 mg, Syrup and Paediatric Liquid. Normal therapeutic dose.
	I.M.	—	—	—	1 mg	5 mg	10 mg	
Metronidazole	Oral	3	—	—	50 mg	100 mg	200 mg	Tab. 200 mg. Dose for Giardiasis 5-day course. Dose for Bacteroides see page 191.
Morphine sulph.	I.M. } S.C.	3	0·15 mg/kg N.B. Avoid if possible	0·2 mg/kg	2 mg	4 mg	8-16 mg	Young children show increased susceptibility to resp. depression. Antidote —Nalorphine.
Naloxone HCl	I.M. I.V. S.C.	Single or as req'd	5-10 mcg/kg				400 mcg	Dose for narcotic overdosage. See newborn section page 59.
			According to manufacturer's literature					
Neostigmine bromide	Oral	3		0·35 mg/kg	3·75 mg	7·5 mg	15 mg	Tabs. 15 mg.

	I.M. I.V.	Once	60 mcg/kg	625 mcg	1·25 mg	2·5 mg	
Neostigmine methyl. sulph.							Atropine usually given first.
Niclosamide	Oral	Single dose	—	500 mg	1 g	2 g	Give half dose, then repeat after 1 hour. Purge after 2 hours. Tabs. 500 mg. Tapeworms (Taeniasis).
Nitrazepam	Oral	3	0·25 mg/kg	2·5 mg	5 mg	10 mg	Anticonvulsant dose. Tabs. 5 mg.
Orciprenaline	Oral	4	0·5 mg/kg	5 mg	10 mg	20 mg	Tabs. 20 mg. Syrup.
Pancreatin B.P. 1973	Oral	Total daily dose stated	500 mg/kg Adjust according to response. Before or with feeds.	5 g	10 g	20 g	
Papaveretum	S.C., or I.M.	3	—	2 mg	5 mg	10–15 mg	
Paracetamol	Oral	3	24 mg/kg	240 mg	500 mg	1 g	Tabs. 500 mg. Elixir Paracetamol for infants B.P.C. contains 120 mg in 5 ml.
Paraldehyde	Oral I.M.	Single dose	0·1 ml/kg	1 ml	2 ml	4 ml	Deep I.M. Very painful. Avoid if possible especially in liver disease.
Pemoline	Oral	2	—	10 mg	20 mg	40 mg	Tab. 20 mg. For hyperkinesia. At night for enuresis.
Pentamidine	I.M.	Daily	—	4 mg/kg daily for 10–14 days			For *Pneumocystis carinii* plus Pyrimethamine.
Pentazocine	Oral I.M. I.V.	4 when required	— — —	— 1 mg/kg 500 mcg/kg	25 mg	50 mg 30–60 mg 30–60 mg	Tabs. 25 mg. Caps 50 mg. Inj.
Pethidine	Oral or S.C.	3	1 mg/kg	12·5 mg	25 mg	50 mg	Tabs. 25 mg and 50 mg.

SOME IMPORTANT DRUGS—(Continued)

Drug	Route	Times Daily	DOSE Caution. Read calculation of dosage for children on page 167					Availability and Remarks
			0-2/52 Neonatal	2/52-1 year	1 year	7 years	Adult	
Pheneturide	Oral	Once	—	—	—	50 mg	100 mg	Tabs. quarter-scored 200 mg.
Phenindione	Oral	Once	—	First day 3 mg/kg	37·5 mg	75 mg	150 mg	Loading dose stated. Decrease dose if liver function impaired.
				Second day 2·5 mg/kg	25 mg	50 mg	100 mg	Tabs. 10 mg, 25 mg and 50 mg.
				Thereafter according to Prothrombin time or "Thrombotest". Usual range for an adult 25-150 mg/day.				
Phenobarbitone	Oral	2	—	3 mg/kg	30 mg	30 mg	30-60 mg	Sedative/Anticonvulsant dose. Young children more tolerant, hence exception in table. They may show behaviour disorders. See page 159.
	I.M.	As req'd	—	6 mg/kg	60 mg	60 mg	60-120 mg	Anticonvulsant dose.
Phenoperidine	I.V. or S.C.	3	—	20 mcg/kg	250 mcg	500 mcg	1 mg	Analgesic dose.
	I.V. or S.C.	Single	—	100 mcg/kg	1 mg	2 mg	4 mg	Resp. Depressant dose. For patients on respirators only.
Phentolamine	I.V. I.M. S.C.	Once	—	0·1 mg/kg	1·25 mg	2·5 mg	5 mg	Test for phaeochromocytoma.
Phenytoin	Oral	3	—	3 mg/kg	30 mg	50 mg	100 mg	Tabs. 100 mg, 50 mg. Suspension 30 mg/5 ml. For single daily maint. dose see page 159.
	I.V. or I.M.	As req'd	—	5 mg/kg	50 mg	100 mg	200 mg	In Status Epilepticus.

Drug	Route	Frequency						Notes
Pholcodine	Oral	3 or 4	—	0·1 mg/kg	1 mg	2 mg	5 mg	Pholcodine Linctus, Strong B.P.C. contains 10 mg/5 ml. Pholcodine Linctus B.P.C. contains 5 mg/5 ml.
Phytomenadione (vit. K_1)	Oral or I.M.	—		0·3 mg/kg	3 mg	5 mg	10 mg	Inj. 10 mg or 1 mg.
Piperazine hydrate	Oral	Twice	—	25 mg/kg	250 mg	500 mg	1 g	Threadworm—7 day course ⎱ see page 79.
	Oral	Single	—	100 mg/kg	1 g	2 g	5 g	Roundworm—single dose treatment ⎰
Potassium chloride	Oral	3 or 4		50 mg/kg 0·5-1 mmol/kg	500 mg 6·5 mmol	1 g 13 mmol	2 g 26 mmol	Maintenance for I.V. therapy, see page 48. 1 g KCl = 13 mmol.K^+ Eff. Tab. 500 mg. Liq. 1 mmol/ml.
Potassium gluconate	Oral	3		150 mg/kg	1·5 g	3 g	6 g	1 g Pot. Gluc. = 4·2 mmol.K^+
Pot. effervescent Tabs. B.P.C. 1 Tab. = 6·5 mmol K^+	Oral	3		Dissolve 1 Tab. in 10 ml give 1 ml/kg	1 Tab.	2 Tabs.	4 Tabs.	N.B. This palatable alternative does not contain any chloride. Continued use may lead to hypochloraemic alkalosis.
Primaquine as base	Oral	Daily for 14 days		375 mcg/kg	3·75 mg	7·5 mg	15 mg	Coated tab. containing 7·5 mg base. Unstable in liq. form. For eradication of P. vivax following 3-day course of Chloroquine.
Primidone	Oral	2		6 mg/kg	62·5 mg	125 mg	250-375 mg	Scored tabs. 250 mg. Susp. 250 mg/5 ml. Converts to Phenobarb. in body. See page 158.
Probenecid	Oral	4		—	Over 2 yrs, 25 mg/kg initially then 10 mg/kg		500 mg	Tab. 250 mg. Adjunct to Penicillin therapy.
Prochlorperazine	Oral	3		0·125 mg/kg	1·25 mg	2·5 mg	5 mg	Antiemetic dose given. I.M.—half stated dose. Rectal—double stated dose. Tabs. 5 mg, 25 mg. Suppositories 5 mg, 25 mg.
Procyclidine	Oral	3		—	—	1·25 mg	2·5 mg	Anti-Parkinson effect. Adjust dose according to response. Tabs. 5 mg.

13A

SOME IMPORTANT DRUGS—(Continued)

Drug	Route	Times Daily	DOSE Caution. Read calculation of dosage for children on page 167					Availability and Remarks
			0-2/52 Neonatal	2/52-1 year	1 year	7 years	Adult	
Promethazine HCl	Oral or I.M.	3	—	—	15 mg	25 mg	25-50 mg	Tabs. 10 mg, 25 mg. Syrup 5 mg/5 ml.
Propantheline bromide	Oral I.M., or I.V.	3	—	—	—	7·5 mg	15 mg	In nocturnal enuresis, single dose may be doubled. Tabs. 15 mg.
Propranolol	Oral / I.V.	3	— / —	1 mg/kg / —	10 mg / 0·3 mg	20 mg / 0·5 mg	40 mg / 1 mg	May be doubled if necessary. Tabs. 10 mg, 40 mg, 80 mg. Initial dose stated. Give stated dose over 1 minute and repeat at 2 minute intervals until desired response or 5 × stated dose achieved. I.V. dose halved for patients under anaesthesia.
Protamine sulph.	I.V.	—	Slowly 1 mg (0·1 ml) for each 100 units Heparin to maximum of 50 mg.					Inj. 10 mg/ml.
Pyrimethamine	Oral	Once	—	—	6·25 mg	12·5 mg	25 mg	Scored tab. 25 mg. Elixir. For Toxoplasmosis 12 day course plus Sulphonamides in full dosage for 28 days with Folinic Acid supplement. For Pneumocystis carinii 12 day course plus Pentamidine. For malarial suppression same dose weekly.
Quinine HCl.	I.V.	12 hrly	5-10 mg/kg Slow I.V. inf. over 4 hours at conc. 50-100 mg/100 ml					For cerebral malaria, until oral therapy possible. Use the lower dose if fits, etc. occur during therapy.
Reserpine	Oral / I.M.	Once / Once	— / —	— / —	20 mcg/kg / 75 mcg/kg May repeat in 12 hours		500 mcg	Tabs. 100 mcg, 250 mcg, 1 mg. Max dose 2·5 mg/day for adult. For Hypertensive crises.
Salbutamol	Oral	3 or 4	—	0·1 mg/kg	1 mg	2 mg	4 mg	Tabs. 2 mg, 4 mg, 8 mg (long-acting) and Syrup.

	Route	Once at night	—	1·5 g	3 g	6 g	
Senna standardised	Oral		—	—			1 leve teaspoonful = 3 g granules = 2 Tabs.
Sodium Valproate	Oral	2	—	10–15 mg/kg			Tab. 200 mg. Syrup 200 mg in 5 ml.
Spironolactone	Oral	4	—	0·6 mg/kg	6·25 mg	12·5 mg	25 mg	Tabs. 25 mg scored.
Sulthiame	Oral	3	—	5 mg/kg	50 mg	100 mg	200 mg	50 mg and 200 mg tabs. Suspension.
Terbutaline	Oral / S.C.	3 / up to 4	—	150 mcg/kg / 5 mcg/kg	1·5 mg / 50 mcg	3 mg / 100 mcg	5 mg / 250 mcg	Tabs. 5 mg and. Syrup.
Thiabendazole	Oral	2	—	25 mg/kg	25 mg/kg		1·5 g	Tabs. 500 mg. Whipworm see page 79.
Thiopentone sod.	Rectal	—	—	25 mg/kg	250 mg	500 mg	1 g	Basal araesthetic dose.
Thyroxine	Oral	Once	12·5 mcg	25 mcg	50 mcg	100 mcg	Initial dose stated. Increase dose at 2/52 intervals according to response. Tabs. 50, 100 mcg.
Trimeprazine tart.	Oral	3	0·25 mg/kg	2·5 mg	5 mg	10 mg	Antipruritic dose. Tabs. 10 mg and Syrup. S'ngle premed. dose is about 10 times sta'ed dose.
Vincristine	I.V.		For leukaemia see page 126.				
Viprynium	Oral	Once	—	75 mg	150 mg	300 mg	Single dose treatment. Threadworm. Tabs. 50 mg and suspension.
Vitamins Compound High potency	I.V.	Once	1 ml	2·5 ml	5 ml	10 ml	Dose stated is total volume from ampoules 1 end 2 mixed before use.
Warfarin	Oral	Once	—	0·75 mg/kg	First day 7·5 mg / 15 mg	27 mg	Loading dose stated. Decrease dose if liver function impaired. Tabs. 1 mg, 3 mg and 5 mg.

Second day No treatment

Thereafter according to Prothrombin time or "Thrombotest". Daily maintenance dose is approximately 1/5 of loading dose.

[NOTES]

XII

ANTIBIOTIC AND CHEMOTHERAPY

GENERAL CONSIDERATIONS

Choice of agent. Before antibiotic treatment is started it is important to obtain an appropriate specimen, such as pus, CSF, blood, urine, pleural fluid, throat swab, etc., in order to determine bacterial sensitivities, see page 77 on management of PUO. In the meantime the infant if ill should be given a suitable antibiotic or combination such as penicillin and an aminoglycoside. If meningitis is suspected or proved the initial treatment might well consist of chloramphenicol, sulphadiazine and penicillin or ampicillin (400 mg/kg/day) by continuous I.V. drip. In the very ill child with osteomyelitis intravenous hydrocortisone in addition to selected antibiotics yields better results.

When the organism has been isolated and its sensitivities determined, suitable drugs can be prescribed, bearing in mind that on occasion combinations of drugs may not only act synergistically but also may delay the emergence of resistant organisms. In general those with the most bactericidal action and narrowest spectrum for the desired effect should be selected, see page 193.

Route

The oral route in general is to be preferred unless contra-indicated by vomiting, diarrhoea or the need quickly to obtain a high blood level. Other factors needing consideration are the blood-brain barrier (page 194) and urinary concentration and reaction.

During Therapy

The mouth must be inspected daily for thrush and where this is present abandonment of broad-spectrum antibiotic treatment may have to be considered.

Vitamin supplements especially the B group and K must be administered when broad-spectrum drugs are used for more than a few days.

Watch for side-effects such as:

Rashes with penicillin, semi-synthetic penicillins especially ampicillin and streptomycin.

187

Eighth nerve affection with streptomycin, kanamycin, gentamicin and tobramycin.

Blood dyscrasias with chloramphenicol.

Gastro-intestinal upsets and superinfection with fungi or resistant staphylococci with tetracyclines and chloramphenicol.

Albuminuria and renal lesions with colistin and polymyxin B and when aminoglycosides are combined with certain diuretics or cephalosporins.

Jaundice with erythromycin estolate.

Tetracyclines—Caution: tooth staining in children under 8 years, see page 192.

Special risks in the *newborn*, see page 71.

Duration of Treatment

In acute infections treatment should be continued until the patient has been afebrile for at least 48 hours. Relapsing conditions such as deep-seated staphylococcal infections, actinomycosis, syphilis, and subacute bacterial endocarditis need special consideration and treatment for several weeks.

Prolonged prophylaxis with penicillin is indicated in acute rheumatism, and in children under 12 years who have had splenectomy.

Interest of the Community

Constant vigilance should be maintained for the emergence of resistant strains and medical staff should discipline themselves in the use of antibiotics.

PRINCIPAL ANTIBIOTIC AND CHEMOTHERAPEUTIC AGENTS

Drug	Route	Times Daily	DOSE — Caution. Read calculation of dosage for children on page 167.					Availability and Remarks
			0-2/52 Neonatal	2-52/1 year	1 year	7 years	Adult	
Amoxycillin	Oral	3	62·5 mg	—	125 mg	250 mg	500 mg	Cap. 250 mg and Syrup.
Amphotericin B	I.V.		—	250 units/kg administered by slow intravenous infusion over a period of 6 hours.	2500 units	5000 units	10,000 units	Initial dose stated. Increase gradually up to maximum of 4 × stated dose, depending on toxicity. Given every 2 days. N.B. Special diluent.
	Oral	4	50-100 mg					Oral thrush. Tabs. 100 mg. Susp. 100 mg/ml. Lozenges 10 mg.
Ampicillin	Oral I.M. or I.V.	4	62·5 mg		125 mg	250 mg	500 mg	Meningitis dose = 400 mg/kg/day by continuous I.V. for 10 days. Tabs. 125 mg. Caps. 250 mg. Syrup. Adult -/T dose 20 mg.
Carbenicillin	I.M. or I.V.	4	50 mg/kg		500 mg	1 g	2 g	Dose may be quadrupled I.V. in severe infections. Use concurrently with Probenecid. Adult I/T 40 mg.
Cephazolin	I.M or I.V.	4	—	25 mg/kg	250 mg	500 mg	1 g	
Cephalexin	Oral	4	12 mg/kg		125 mg	250 mg	500 mg	Caps. 2·0 mg and 500 mg. Susp.
Cephaloridine	I.M.	2 or 3	12 mg/kg		125 mg	250 mg	500 mg	Adult I/T dose, 50 mg.
Cephradine	Oral I.M. or I.V.	4	12 mg/kg		125 mg	250 mg	500 mg	Cap. 250 mg and 500 mg. Syrup.
Chloramphenicol	Oral I.M. or I.V.	4	Avoid	12 mg/kg	125 mg	250 mg	500 mg	Caution—Aplastic anaemia. I/T dose 1-2 mg daily. Caps. 250 mg. Suspension.

PRINCIPAL ANTIBIOTIC AND CHEMOTHERAPEUTIC AGENTS —(Continued)

Drug	Route	Times Daily	DOSE Caution. Read calculation of dosage for children on page 167.					Availability and Remarks
			0-2/52 Neonatal	2/52-1 year	1 year	7 years	Adult	
Clindamycin	Oral	3 or 4	—	37·5 mg	75 mg	150 mg	30 mg	Caps. 75 mg and 150 mg. Susp.
Colistin sulphomethate (Polymyxin E)	I.M or I.V.	3	—	25,000 units/kg	250,000 units	500,000 units	1,000,000 units	I/T dose 500–1000 units/kg.
Co-trimoxazole	Oral	2 Proph. Night	Avoid Avoid	4 mg/kg 2 mg/kg	40 mg 20 mg	80 mg 40 mg	160 mg 80 mg	Doses stated in terms of Trimethoprim. Adult tabs. Trimethoprim 80 mg and Sulphamethoxazole 400 mg. Paediatric tabs. Trimethoprim 20 mg and Sulphamethoxazole 100 mg. Susp. 40 mg/5 ml and 80 mg/5 ml.
Erythromycin	Oral I.V.	4	12 mg/kg	12 mg/kg	125 mg	250 mg	500 mg	Tabs. 100 mg and 250 mg. Suspension Lactobionate I.V. See page 188 for salts and possible jaundice.
Erythromycin ethylsuccinate	I.M.	3	2·5 mg/kg	2·5 mg/kg	25 mg	50 mg	100 mg	Painful.
Flucloxacillin and Cloxacillin	Oral I.M. or I.V.	4	62·5 mg	62·5 mg	125 mg	250 mg	500 mg	Flucloxacillin better absorbed orally. Caps. 250 mg. Syrup. Adult I/T dose 10 mg.
Flucytosine	Oral	4	—	150–200 mg/kg/day				Tab. 500 mg. Adjust dose in renal impairment. Antifungal agent.
Fusidic Acid	Oral I.V.	4 3	— —	12·5 mg/kg as Acid 20 mg/kg/24 hrs* as Sod. salt		250 mg Sod. 250 mg	500 mg Sod. 500 mg	Cap. 250 mg (Sod. salt). Susp. 250 mg (Acid) = 175 mg Sod. salt Synergism with Penicillin. See literature. Inj. only I.V., as continuous infusion. *Double this dose under 1 year.
Gentamicin	I.M.	3	3 mg/kg 12-hrly	2 mg/kg				1st dose ONLY 3 mg/kg. 8th Nerve Toxicity. Assess blood levels. I.V. same dose by bolus only.

Drug	Route	Times daily						Remarks
Isoniazid (I.N.A.H.)	Oral	Once	—	7·5 mg/kg	75 mg	150 mg	300 mg	Tab. 50 mg and 100 mg. Pyridoxine may be given concurrently. See combined P.A.S. and I.N.A.H. preparations.
Kanamycin	I.M.	2		7·5 mg/kg	75 mg	200 mg	500 mg	Nephrotoxic, 8th Nerve Toxicity.
Lincomycin	Oral	3	—	12 mg/kg	125 mg	250 mg	500 mg	Double dose in severe infection. Caps. 500 mg. Syrup, Amps. 600 mg/2 ml. I.V. as continuous infusion.
	I.M. I.V. }	3	—	10–15 mg/kg	150 mg	300 mg	600 mg	
Metronidazole	Oral	3	—		7 mg/kg		400 mg	Tab. 200 mg, 400 mg. Suppos. 500 mg, 1g. For Bacteroides treatment 7-day course.
	Rectal	3	—		500 mg		1 g	
Nalidixic acid	Oral	4	Avoid	25 mg/kg	250 mg	500 mg	1 g	Tabs. 500 mg. Suspension. Reduce for prophylaxis.
Neomycin	Oral	4		12 mg/kg	125 mg	250 mg	500 mg	Not absorbed. Tabs. 500 mg. Syrup.
Nitrofurantoin	Oral	4		2·5 mg/kg	25 mg	50 mg	100 mg	Tabs. 50 mg and 100 mg. Suspension. Prophylaxis half stated dose at night.
Nystatin	Oral	4	Oral thrush 100,000 units on tongue for local action.					Oral susp. and Tabs. ½ mega. Little absorption.
P.A.S.	Oral	2		150 mg/kg	1·5 g	3 g	5 g	
P.A.S. and I.N.A.H. combined	Oral	2	Up to a max. of 30 kg body weight give PAS 150 mg/kg & INAH 3·75 mg/kg.					Sachets containing either PAS 2 g & INAH 50 mg or PAS 6 g & INAH 150 mg.
Penicillin G.	I.M.	2		15 mg/kg	150 mg (¼ mega)	300 mg (½ mega)	600 mg (1 mega)	Crystalline or Benzyl Penicillin 1 mega unit = 600 mg. Give same dose 6-hourly in severe infection. Adult I/T dose = 6 mg.
Penicillin procaine inj.	I.M. only	Once		0·05 ml/kg	0·5 ml	1 ml	2 ml	300,000 units/ml.
Penicillin prolonged action	I.M. only	—		¼ vial every 3 days		½ vial every 3 days	1 vial every 3 days	Each vial contains: Penicillin G. 300 mg, Procaine Pen. 250 mg, Benethamine Pen. 475 mg.

PRINCIPAL ANTIBIOTIC AND CHEMOTHERAPEUTIC AGENTS—(Continued)

Drug	Route	Times Daily	DOSE Caution. Read calculation of dosage for children on page 167.					Availability and Remarks
			0-2/52 Neonatal	2/52-1 year	1 year	7 years	Adult	
Penicillin V, Phenoxymethyl Penicillin	Oral	4	62.5 mg		125 mg	250 mg	500 mg	Tabs. 125 mg and 250 mg. Syrup. 124 mg/5 ml.
Rifampicin	Oral	Daily	—	15 mg/kg	150 mg	300 mg	600 mg	Cap. 150 mg and 300 mg. Susp. 100 mg/5 ml.
Streptomycin	I.M.	Once	Avoid	25 mg/kg	250 mg	500 mg	1 g	Suggested dose if for T.B. therapy. For short-term therapy dose may be increased by 50%. I/T dose 1 mg/kg/day.
SULPHONAMIDES								
Phthalylsulphathiazole	Oral	4	Avoid	50 mg/kg	500 mg	1 g	2 g	Not absorbed. Tabs. 500 mg. Suspension.
Sulphadimidine / Sulphadiazine	Oral / I.M. or I.V.	4	Avoid	25 mg/kg	250 mg	500 mg	1 g	Dose doubled in severe infection. Tabs. 500 mg. Mixture 500 mg/5 ml.
Sulphasalazine	Oral	4	—	—	250 mg	500 mg	1 g	Ulcerative colitis. 500 mg Tabs.
Tetracycline HCl. and Oxytetracycline	Oral / I.M.	4 / 3	6·25 mg/kg / 2·5 mg/kg		62·5 mg / 25 mg	125 mg / 50 mg	250 mg / 100 mg	Tabs. 250 mg. Syrup. Tetracycline with Procaine Inj. B.P. Caution. Tooth-staining in children under 8 years.
	I.V.	4			62·5 mg	125 mg	250 mg	
Tobramycin	I.M.	3	3 mg/kg 12-hourly	2 mg/kg				8th Nerve Toxicity. Assess blood levels. I.V. same dose by bolus inj. only.

ANTIBIOTICS FOR SPECIFIC BACTERIA (SUBJECT TO LABORATORY TESTS)

	Penicillin	Ampicillin/Amoxycillin	Flucloxacillin	Cephaloridine	Cephalexin	Carbenicillin	Erythromycin	Lincomycin/Clindamycin	Fusidic Acid	Sulphonamides	Co-trimoxazole	Tetracycline†	Chloramphenicol	Streptomycin	Kanamycin	Gentamicin/Tobramycin	Colomycin
Staph. aureus*—penicillin sensitive	1	0	0	2	2	0	2	2	2	0	2	2	0	2	2	2	×
Staph. aureus*—penicillin resistant	×	×	1	2	2	×	2	2	2	0	2	2	0	2	2	2	×
Streptococci and pneumococci	1	0	0	2	2	0	2	2	0	0	2	2	0	×	×	×	×
Str. faecalis	0	1	0	×	×	×	2	×	0	×	2	2	0	×	×	×	×
Esch. coli	×	1	×	2	2	0	×	×	×	0	2	2	0	2	2	2	0
Klebsiellae	×	0	×	1	1	2	×	×	×	0	2	2	0	2	2	2	0
Proteus	×	1	×	2	2	2	×	×	×	0	2	×	0	2	2	2	×
Pseudomonas	×	×	×	×	×	1	×	×	×	×	×	×	×	×	×	1	2
Other Gram-negatives	0	2	×	0	2	0	×	×	×	2	1	2	×	0	0	0	0
Clostridia	1	0	0	2	0	0	2	2	0	×	×	2	0	×	×	×	×
Listeria	2	1	×	0	×	0	2	0	0	0	0	2	0	0	0	0	×
Haemophilus—other than meningitis	0	1	×	×	×	0	2	×	×	0	2	0	1	0	0	0	×
Bacteroides	0	×	×	×	×	×	2	1	0	0	0	0	2	×	×	×	×
Bordetella pertussis	×	1	×	×	×	0	0	×	×	×	×	2	2	×	×	×	0

* most strains penicillin-resistant.
† tetracycline should be avoided below age 8 years.
1 = first line
2 = second line
0 = not usually recommended
× = inactive

ANTIBIOTICS AND THE BLOOD-BRAIN BARRIER

	Penetration of inflamed meninges	*Daily intrathecal dose in neonates**
Sulphonamides	Good	—
Co-trimoxazole		—
Chloramphenicol		(1–2 mg into abscess cavities)
Tetracycline	Adequate from	—
Erythromycin	intensive I.V.	—
Lincomycin	therapy	—
Penicillin G		1500 units
Ampicillin		2·5 mg
Flucloxacillin	Poor	2·5 mg
Carbenicillin		5 mg
Cephaloridine		5 mg
Gentamicin		1 mg
Kanamycin	Very poor	1–2 mg
Streptomycin		1 mg/kg
Colistin		500 units/kg

* Intrathecal dose for older children given under main antibiotic section.

XIII

CORTICOSTEROIDS

GENERAL CONSIDERATIONS

THE steroids secreted by the adrenal cortex are divided into three groups—the mineralocorticoids, the glucocorticoids and the anabolic steroids.

The starting dosage of some synthetic steroids in these three groups which are now in common usage is given on pages 199 and 200. Steroid toxicity can be minimised by giving 48 hours' dosage as a single dose on alternate days. Corticotrophin (ACTH) is used when it is desired to stimulate the patient's adrenal cortex.

PRECAUTIONS IN TREATMENT

In hospital, weights and blood pressures should be recorded each day. Potassium supplements are not needed if the child is taking a full diet. Careful watch for signs of infection should be maintained and antibiotics used more readily than usual if infection is suspected. All the infections of childhood have been shown to produce severe reactions in children having corticosteroid therapy. When an infection, or other stress such as a surgical operation, is encountered in a child, the maintenance dose of the drug, if small, should be increased $2\frac{1}{2}$–5 times. When the drug is stopped the adrenal cortex may take an indefinite time to recover and therefore, during the following two years any infection should be covered by the equivalent of 50 mg of cortisone daily.

Scheme of steroid cover before, during and after operation

For children who have received steroids in prolonged or heavy dosage whether oral, systemic or by rectum at any time during the previous two years the following scheme is suggested. If the daily dose has been more than 100 mg of cortisone or its equivalent, double the amounts pre- and postoperatively, returning to the previous dose on the fourth day.

12 hours before operation: 100 mg cortisone I.M.

1 hour before operation: 100 mg cortisone I.M.

First 24 hours post-operatively: 50 mg cortisone by mouth 6-hourly or 100 mg I.M. 12-hourly.

Second 24 hours post-operatively:	50 mg cortisone 8-hourly by mouth or 75 mg I.M. 12-hourly.
Third 24 hours post-operatively:	50 mg cortisone 12-hourly by mouth or I.M. if necessary.
Fourth 24 hours post-operatively:	25 mg cortisone 12-hourly by mouth or I.M. if necessary.

During operation and for 24 hours afterwards hydrocortisone for intravenous use must be *immediately available* in the theatre or at the bedside.

OUTPATIENT CARE

After the patient's discharge from hospital the family doctor and the parents must be instructed that (1) the drug must be taken exactly as prescribed, (2) that the dose must be raised during infection or stress to an equivalent of about 50 mg cortisone per day.

In nearly all cases, and certainly when the dose used is large, regular attendance in the clinic should be required. Weight, height, and blood pressure must be recorded at each visit. An X-ray estimate of vertebral bone-density and of bone age should be made every year.

Parents of children who are non-immune to varicella and measles should be warned of the potential hazards and advised to report any contact immediately so that appropriate protective measures (pages 82 and 83) can be taken.

A card giving details of therapy should be issued to all patients with advice to carry it at all times.

PRINCIPAL STEROIDS AND INITIAL DOSAGE

GLUCOCORTICOIDS

In treatment of conditions amenable to glucocorticoid therapy, Prednisolone/Prednisone are the drugs of choice. Parenteral therapy is usually given as Hydrocortisone Hemisuccinate for rapid action or with the Acetate Suspension I.M. for depot therapy.

Drug	Route	Times Daily	DOSE — Caution. Read calculation of dosage for children on page 167.					Availability and Remarks
			0-2/52 Neonatal	2/52-1 year	1 year	7 years	Adult	
Prednisolone	Oral	3	0·7 mg/kg		7·5 mg	15 mg	30 mg	Tabs. 5 mg and 1 mg. Leukaemia dose, see page 125.
Prednisone			Dose for Idiopathic Nephrotic Syndrome 60 mg/m²/day. Max. 80 mg/day.					
Hydrocortisone Hemisuccinate	I.V. I.M. }		All ages—Pharmacological doses 50-100 mg repeatable 6-hourly.					
Hydrocortisone Acetate	I.M.	Once	3 mg/kg		30 mg	62·5 mg	125 mg	I.M. absorption takes 48-72 hours.
ACTH (Corticotrophin) Gel.} Zn.}	I.M.	Once	1 i.u./kg		10 i.u.	20 i.u.	40 i.u.	Long-acting. ACTH test, see page 143.

Equivalent (anti-inflammatory) doses of other steroids are shown below. These figures also correspond with tablet strength.

Cortisone 25 mg	Hydrocortisone 20 mg
Prednisone 5 mg	Methylprednisolone 5 mg
Triamcinolone 5 mg	Dexamethasone 0·75 mg
Betamethasone 0·5 mg	

PRINCIPAL STEROIDS AND INITIAL DOSAGE—(Continued)

MINERALOCORTICOIDS   Physiological replacement doses.

Drug	Route	Times Daily	DOSE — Caution. Read calculation of dosage for children on page 167				Availability and Remarks
			0-2/52 Neonatal	2/52-1 year	1 year	7 years	Adult	
Fludrocortisone acetate	Oral	Once	—	5 mcg/kg	50 mcg	100 mcg	200 mcg	Tabs. 100 mcg.

Specific treatment for Addisonian crisis.

Hydrocortisone Hemisuccinate I.V. 50–100 mg. Same dose I.M. at same time and 8-hourly for 24 hours, then 12-hourly for 24 hours.

ANABOLIC STEROIDS

Drug	Route	Times Daily	DOSE — Caution. Read calculation of dosage for children on page 167				Availability and Remarks
			0-2/52 Neonatal	2/52-1 year	1 year	7 years	Adult	
Methandienone	Oral	Once	—	0·04 mg/kg	0·4 mg	1·25 mg	2·5 mg	5 mg Tabs.

N.M.B

INDEX

Acid-base bnlaace, 139
Acidosis, 49
ACTH test, 143
Adrenal-pituitary tests, 141
Adrenocortical crisis, 95
Adrenogenital syndrome, 95
Alkalosis, 52
Amniocentesis and fetal diagnosis, 156
Anaemia, 25
Analysis of milk formulae, 19
Antibiotic therapy, 187
Antibiotics and blood/brain barrier, 194
Antibiotics, side-effects, 187
  for specific bacteria, 193
Anticonvulsants, 159
Asthma, 93
Astrup readings, 139

Bacterial sensitivities, 193
Battered baby, 91, 153
Beriberi, 28
Biochemical investigations, 139
  special tests, 146
  standards, 137, 138
Blood transfusion, 133
Blood volume, 133
Bone age, 8–10
Breast feeding, 17
Bronchiolitis, 92
Burns, 109

Calcium, daily needs, 18
Calories, daily needs, 18
Candidal infections, 81
Carbohydrate, daily needs, 18
Cardiac arrest, 107
Cardiac emergencies, 103
Cardioversion, 108
Caustic burns, 118
Centile tables for growth, 11, 12
Cerebral oedema, 121
Chromosomal analysis, 155

Coagulation investigations, 132
Collapse, acute, in infancy, 94
Coma, 90
Convulsions, 90, 157
Coroner, reporting to, 159
Corticosterolds, 197–200
Cryoprecipitate, 127

Daily intakes for healthy children, 18
Dehydration, 48, 89
Development, infancy and childhood, 5, 6
Diabetes insipidus, 145
Diabetes mellitus, 100–103
Diets, 38–41
Digoxin dosage, 105
Disseminated intravascular coagulation, 127
Dosage calculation, 167–169
Dwarfism, 141–144

Electrolytes, 47–53
  composition of alimentary fluids, 50
Encephalitis, 90
Epiglottitis, 91
Epilepsy, 157
Exchange transfusion, 72

Feeding, healthy children, 17
  sick infant, 21
Feeds, normal, 19
  special, 31–37
Fits, 90, 157
Fluid, daily needs, 18
  insensible loss, 98
Fresh frozen plasma, 127, 128, 133

G-6-PD deficiency, 130
Galactosaemia, test, 146
Gammaglobulin, virus infections, 83

Gangliosidosis, 146
Gastro-enteritis, 89
Genetic counselling, 155
Glucagon test, 140
Glucose tolerance, 139
Glycogen storage disease, 141, 146
Gonadal function, 141
Growth charts, 4, 11, 12

Haematological, disorders, 125
  values, 133
Haemoglobinopathies, 129–130
Haemolytic disease of newborn, 71
Haemolytic-uraemic syndrome, 96
Haemorrhagic disorders, 127
Head injury, 91
Heart disease, 103
Homocystinuria, 146
Hypernatraemia, 51
Hypertensive crises, 99
Hypoglycaemia, investigation of,
  140

Immunisation schedule, 84
Immunity and the newborn, 83
Incubation periods, 78
Infectious disease, 78
Inquest, advice on attending, 160
Insensible fluid loss, 98
Insulin, dosage, 101–103
  sensitivity test, 142
Intrathecal therapy, 127, 170, 194
Intravenous therapy, 47
Iodine deficiency, 28
Iron content of milk, 19
  daily needs, 18
  deficiency, 25
Isolation periods, 78

Ketovite, 36

Lesch–Nyhan syndrome, 146
Leucine sensitivity test, 140
Leukaemia, 125–127
Lipidaemias, 146
Lumbar puncture warning, 90, 91

Magnesium, daily needs, 18
Malabsorption, 147
Malaria, 77, 81, 90
Meningitis, neonatal, 67
  other, 90
Metabolic disease, 146, 157
Metachromatic leucodystrophy, 147
Milk formulae, 19
  special preparations, 29–33
Mineral and vitamin supplements,
  20, 29, 36
Mixed feeding of infants, 17
Mucopolysaccharidoses, 147

Needs, daily, 18
Newborn, antibiotics, 74
  apnoea, 59, 66
  cardiac conditions, 65, 103
  cerebral symptoms, 67
  examination of, 60
  haemolytic disease, 71
  hypocalcaemia, 68
  hypoglycaemia, 68
  hypomagnesaemia, 68
  hypothermia, 63
  infant of diabetic mother, 64
  infections, 73
  intestinal obstruction, 69
  intra-uterine weight chart, 61
  jaundice, 70
  light for dates, 64
  low birth weight, 63
  major symptoms, 65
  maturity assessment, 62
  meningitis, 67
  respiratory distress, 65
  resuscitation, 59
  shock, 69
  special problems, 63
  vomiting, 69
Non-accidental injury, 91, 153
Nuclear sexing, 155
Nutrition, 17
  parenteral, 52
Nutritional disorders, 23

Oedema, cerebral, 121
Oesophageal atresia, 69
Operation and steroids, 197
Organic acidaemias, 147
Osseous centres, 8–10

Parasites, 79, 80
Paroxysmal tachycardia, 104
Pellagra, 28
Phenylketonuria test, 147
Pituitary-adrenal function, 141
Plasma, fresh frozen, 127, 128, 133
Poisoning, 113–121
 alcohol, 118
 amphetamine, 118
 atropine, 118
 household products, 118
 iron, 116
 lead, 120
 paracetamol, 116
 paraffin, 119
 paraquat, 119
 phenothiazines, 117
 plants, 120
 psychotrophic drugs, 117
 salicylates, 115
 tricyclics, 117
Porphyria, 147
Potassium, daily needs, 18, 47
 overdosage, 48
Prescribing, 167
Protein, daily needs, 18
 energy deficiency, 26
Protozoal infections, 80
Pyrexia of uncertain origin, 77

Quarantine, 78

Renal, dialysis, indication for, 99
 failure, 96
 function tests, 144

Respiratory emergencies, 91
Rhesus incompatibility, 71

Sensitivities, bacterial, 193
Skull circumference, 11, 12
Sodium, daily needs, 18, 47
Steroid dosage, 197–200
Stridor, 91
Surface area nomogram, 168
Suxamethonium sensitivity, 147
Sweat test, 148, 149
Synthetic foods and vitamin supplements, 29, 36

Tachycardia, paroxysmal, 104
Tetanus prophylaxis, 85
Thalassaemia, 129
Thyroid function, 143
Transfusion rates, 133
Tube feeding, 22
Typhoid (enteric), 77, 78

Virus infections, 82
 and the newborn, 83
Vitamin and mineral supplements, 20, 29, 36

Warning signs at different ages, 7
Weaning, 17
Weight tables, 11, 12
Wilson's disease, 147
Worms, 79–80